Dosha for Life

Dosha for Life

*A Contemporary Examination of the
Ancient Ayurvedic Science of Self-healing*

Linda Bretherton

and

Jim Whitham

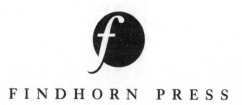

FINDHORN PRESS

First published by Findhorn Press 2007

ISBN: 978-1-84409-109-6

British Library Cataloguing-in-Publication Data.
A catalogue record for this book is available from the British Library.

Edited by Jane Engel
Cover design by Damian Keenan
Layout by Pam Bochel
Printed and bound by WS Bookwell, Finland

1 2 3 4 5 6 7 8 9 10 11 12 13 12 11 10 09 08 07

Published by
Findhorn Press
305A The Park,
Findhorn, Forres
Scotland IV36 3TE

Tel 01309 690582
Fax 01309 690036
email: info@findhornpress.com
www.findhornpress.com

Contents

Chapter 1

A Journey into Ayurveda

What is Ayurveda? Directly translated Ayurveda means 'The Science of Life.' It is one of the oldest forms of healing the world has known, with its origins dating back 5000 years to the Vedic sages who lived in that part of the Asian subcontinent now known as India, and is one of the most profound health practices in the world. Ayurveda is a system of preventative healthcare and healing and is also a philosophy for living. It cures not by simply treating the symptoms but by removing the causes of disease and by guiding us to balance the physical and spiritual elements of our lives. Within Ayurveda the objective is to achieve balance as an individual whose emotional life, intake of food, output of energy and whose attention to the daily act of living is also extended to take in the wider concept of a harmonious universe.

Recent years have seen a rise in popularity for many holistic health disciplines and Ayurveda is no exception, with steadily increasing numbers of practitioners, schools and opportunities for therapies. However something is being ignored in many of the variations of treatments and teachings now becoming available. With the western outlook, which inclines towards quick fixes and a prescriptive solution, a core premise is in danger of being lost. We are holistic beings who reflect and react to the whole experience of life around us. The central Ayurvedic concept of balance and harmony between all living things is as fundamental today as it was 5000 years ago. Within Ayurveda the earth is seen to be an interrelated whole, a vast living organism. We humans share the same atomic and molecular structures and the same building blocks as all life forms and what happens to one part affects the whole. Our world is a wonderful living entity; the atmosphere that we live in, the oxygen, the weather systems, the natural resources, the earth and the sea, the animal and plant life are all connected. Changes to the seasons, to the natural and built environment create cross currents of influence that affect everything around us. Loss of this sense of connection to our environment has led to the malaise that is damaging the planet and most human relationships.

In the steady acceleration of our pace of life we have become disconnected from our sources. We have forgotten how to be aware, how to respond with intuition to our surroundings and how to take care of ourselves. We have become accustomed to taking pills and whole arsenals of chemical supplements, and we have buried the intuitive responses to health that were once central to our way of life. Searching for outside guidance has become the norm. We are losing touch with the natural rhythms and cycles of nature and with the creative act of living in harmony with these powerful forces.

The thinking mind has enabled mankind to create complex structures, systems and technologies, but is has also created war, slaughter and destruction on a grand scale. On a smaller scale, through thought patterns and behaviour that corrode well-being, we damage and limit ourselves and our loved ones on a daily basis. In our technological age we see increasing evidence of downsizing and restructuring in industry; rising stress levels on workers who take on the jobs of three people with less job security; and depression and a sense of hopelessness in those without work. The disparity between wealth and poverty is brought home forcibly through relentless media channels. The speed of today's society seems to have increased whilst our transport systems have slowed down, national health waiting lists create anxiety in the sick—the list goes on and on. Such stresses and distractions have disconnected us from the most important aspects of life.

Ayurveda teaches us how to rediscover critical knowledge and awareness of the natural forces and rhythms that compliment and strengthen our human experience, through delicious nutrition using natural herbs and spices, through enhanced levels of self awareness involving practical daily activities and through attention to our total environment to bring about radical changes in outlook and in health.

How are we linked to all life forms and to our environment?

Despite all the technological advances in our world and any amount of material success, we are all made from the same elements as ancient people. Progress in science and corresponding levels of human brain activity, of reason and thought have allowed us to develop in particular ways. We have advanced from our ancestors in our capacity to identify and use a wide range of resources, to break the constraints of our immediate surroundings and time zones, and in our use of knowledge. We have vast reservoirs of information at our disposal. Nevertheless this doesn't alter the fact that we are natural beings in a natural world, regardless of any technical advances.

Ayurveda sees the world composed of 5 elements, which are ether/space, air, fire, water and earth. *Each and every living thing is composed of these elements,* which form vital energies that fluctuate according to our state of balance as individuals and the seasons of nature. We consist of trillions of cells that themselves contain the same ingredients as every other living thing, a fact that may be hard to believe, but is nevertheless true. Scientist have known for a long time that things aren't what they seem and that the real differences between things aren't what they are made from but how the basic ingredients are utilised. Life is recognised at the quantum level to consist of pulses of energy that differ in frequency between life forms, "non-living" matter and between different levels of awareness. At the sub-atomic level we have the same ingredients as a flower, or a bird, a rock or a drop of rain. We have the elements of earth, water, fire, air and space within our bodies in the form of acids, enzymes, fluids and tissues. These elements and our human pulse of life are sustained by nutrition in the very broadest sense. We obtain that from food, from our breathing and from the attention we give to ourselves. The quality of attention communicates our intent and we flourish when given the right kind of attention and wither when given the wrong kind.

Challenging assumptions

Contrary to a popular saying, we are not just what we eat; we are also what we think and what we do. Just as importantly, we each have a distinct individual body type that governs our physical and emotional health and outlook and the way we respond to things around us. This body type never changes but may suffer from fluctuations in the way it manifests our state of wellbeing. It helps to underpin our identity and affects our behaviour throughout our lives. We can recognise this fact, work with it to feel and look better, or we can ignore our true nature, fight it and be continually stressed and unhappy. How do we make the best of this natural gift of a body type? Simply by paying attention and getting to know ourselves. **The key factors that influence our quality of life for good or bad are food, exercise and activity, our home and working environments and the way we use our mind and senses. Dramatic changes to our outlook, health and energy happen as a result of what we put into our hearts, minds and bodies. Getting to know ourselves means recognising who and what we are and working with the natural attributes we are born with.**

Our bodies rebuild themselves many times throughout our lifetime. Cells from every organ are renewed by the food that we eat. Every breath we take and every mouthful that we swallow contributes to this building process. Every taste, every sight and smell, in fact every sensory experience connected with food, rebuilds or damages our cells and imprints itself into our emotions and the sensory experience of being alive. From these basic building blocks we create ourselves on an hourly and daily basis. Then our thinking mind continues the process of creation or destruction, through the attitudes we adopt from our upbringing and our relationships. The good and the bad, the healthy and the unhealthy aspects of our lives all originate from the processes that go on within us and from the way we co-operate with our bodies, or alternatively try to fight them into submission.

Body types or Doshas

As people come in so many shapes and sizes, colours and weight, it seems obvious that we shouldn't all eat and do the same things to make us healthy and happy. We are all individuals with different tastes and experiences and there are more variations in people-types than there are Atkins Diets and GI diets and all the other fashions and fads. We see the more extreme visible signs every day when we go to work or go to the shops. We see "thinnies" and "fatties" and some "in-betweenies" and we see redheads and darker swarthier types and short and tall people and all the sizes in between, but they only reveal half the picture. The physical differences can be important clues but they don't tell us about emotional characteristics, about behaviour, why some people never gain weight and others can never shake it off, or why some are constant worriers and others struggle to rouse themselves into action. In another context we might suffer from all kinds of ailments yet— despite the wide range of people-types, the differences in how we react to food, to our surroundings and to each other—we are all treated by the mainstream health industry in broad brush strokes. Even a headache is usually dealt with by a very limited range of options centred on paracetamol or aspirin, blanket-bombing the symptoms and avoiding the cause which could have been anything from anxiety, tiredness, dehydration or reaction to food just to name a few possibilities all of which could be treated by holistic methods.

There are indeed great differences between people, but fortunately there is also a detailed map to guide us through the maze and help us to make sense of what might at first seem to be a random collection of types. There are common factors arising from the five elements of **ether/space, air, fire, water and earth** and these elements form unique balances within each individual to create their body type or dosha. No two people are exactly the same. We all have the same ingredients, but in differing quantities and with Ayurveda we learn how to recognise the balance of elements that form our dosha and how to respond to their dynamics. We will look at this in more detail later.

Body type, attitude and behaviour are all linked. We think, look and act in repeating patterns throughout our lives and this behaviour is always linked to something fundamental within our personality and within our cells at the deepest level, where the five elements are located. In Ayurveda our body type or dosha provides the key to understanding what we are, allowing us to examine and fine-tune our diets and lifestyles to create health, strength and energy for life. We each have a unique collection of experiences and memories that have helped to make us what we are—or at least what we think we are. However, underlying these experiences our dosha is distinct and unchanging, providing us with default patterns from which our responses originate. We may gain or lose weight, change jobs, clothes, hair style and colour, but underneath these superficial differences our dosha and its inherent traits, fixed before we were born, will always govern our initial state of mind and our emotional and physical responses to life. That is not to say we are the victims of our dosha. We can create ourselves to be the best we can be by choosing to learn about and to work with this fundamental natural resource.

Our doshas have clearly defined characteristics and specific nutritional, emotional and spiritual needs. Our preferences for food, colour, tastes, textures, sounds and activities are founded upon this cellular make-up. When we put the wrong kinds of food into our body, when we labour away with thoughts and activities in environments that don't suit us, we may as well be taking poison— on a daily basis. When we remain ignorant of these characteristics we ignore the whole foundation of who we really are. Knowing our dosha helps us to understand that certain kinds of foods are more useful to us than others. We are also better suited to certain sounds, textures, colours, smells, oils and environments. We also react physically and emotionally to the changing seasons and climate in different ways according to our dosha. How we function and behave, how we respond to these elements in our daily lives and the fluctuations in our emotions, are all affected by this metabolic template within us. When we live, eat and do things that go against the best interest of our body type we are actively damaging everything that we are!

So what is a body type? What is it that actually makes a body type or dosha?

There are many factors that determine doshas and we will give you clear guidance in identifying and understanding your own. We have chosen to illustrate this work through three case studies in a unique way that is easy to understand. Each study is typical of one of the three main doshas. In many ways they represent the extremes, since they are unusually high in the qualities of one particular dosha, a rare occurrence, but for this reason they will provide greater clarity to you, the reader. Most people are combinations of the three doshas, one dominant with varying percentages of the other two. As we work through the case studies some of you will immediately begin to recognise your own more obvious physical and emotional qualities and this will be the start of your education. Later you can work through the questionnaires in Appendix A to establish your own unique mix of dosha characteristics.

Ayurveda defines three main doshas created by the energy forces of **ether/space, air, fire, water and earth** within us. *Ether* and *space* are inextricably linked and form one element that is the first universal element from which all life originates. *Ether* constitutes the potential condition for all life, for creation, for action and is within every cell of our bodies. The other elements are in many ways easier to understand when we consider the natural world. *Air* moves, shifting like the wind and creating movement through our bodies. It is the medium through which we receive life-giving oxygen. *Fire* comes in the form of sunlight, generating the plant life, which underpins all life on the planet, and in the form of chemicals and enzymes within the digestive process. *Fire* transforms. *Water* is central to our lives. We are at least 60% water, and it lubricates our cells and transports every essential element our tissues need to survive. *Earth* is the basis of our physical growth and our link to the planet's life cycles spanning millions of years. Each element is present in all of us and we shall describe their function in greater detail in Chapter Two. Each of these forces exists in an unequal balance within each individual and it is that state of dynamic tension that creates our dosha, formed from a combination of the three main doshas. They are known by the

Sanskrit names of **Vata, Pitta and Kapha** and have particular work to do in our bodies. We need them all to function together.

Vata, the most common dosha, consists of the elements of air and ether/space and works with the nervous system to control all body movement, including nutrients and waste. In the mind, Vata is concerned with memory and comparison of information. Air is the breath, which stimulates movement. Ether/space is where the vibration of all vital systems and all creative activity occur. Unlike Pitta and Kapha, which consist of two contrasting and counter-balancing elements, Vata's two elements of ether and air have very similar characteristics and as a consequence Vata types are prone to the typical extremes of behaviour and conditions that we will examine in our case study.

Pitta consists of the elements of fire and water and governs the body's balance of chemical and transforming energies, including the digestion of both food and thought. In the mind, Pitta processes new data and draws conclusions. Fire is the acids and enzymes of the body and the sun's rays that directly affect all life forms and the environment. Water is present in every cell and it can be calm or turbulent. The balance of opposites within Pitta between fire and water is critical and our case study reveals the damaging effects when imbalance occurs between these contrasting elements.

Kapha consists of the elements of earth and water and governs structure, bodily stability, lubrication, and cell structure. In the mind, Kapha provides stability and the ability to grasp single thoughts. The earth is our physical body and is solid and grounding. Water is the fluid present in every cell and mixed with earth can become dense and heavy. When imbalanced these elements combine to bind and weigh down upon Kapha types.

The difference between the three main body types arises then from these combinations of elements. What happens with combinations of the three will be examined in detail later, but it's worth re-stating that aspects of all three types are in each of us, and that some are simply more dominant than others. Each element contains forces essential for the functioning of our bodies.

These doshas form the foundation for all humans and are mirrored in the seasons and cycles of nature. Since the doshas are created by the balance of natural elements in our cells, they never change. Once we grow from a single cell that multiplies in our mother's womb, these characteristics are established. They are our default pattern. As we mature we build a bank of experiences, we are affected by life around us and we may become ill or unhappy, gain or lose weight, hair and common sense, but our essential nature remains. Imbalances occur as a result of events in our lives and our environment, when our inherent characteristics may become exaggerated or extreme, but our essential constitution never changes. The irony is that we hardly ever recognise our essential nature because of the welter of external influences that pour over us and this is where awareness comes into play. As adults we have the ability to choose; we can adapt to our circumstances and create all that is possible within our powers. The secret is to know this essential being within us and to keep it in balance. Our power and creativity arise from this balanced state, which requires attention and daily maintenance. Food is an excellent starting point.

The nourishing elements in our food are the same elements that we are composed of. Our food, which contains the elements of **ether/space, air, fire, water and earth**, has an inheritance that passes on to us in the continual rebuilding process of life. We don't have to think about it because it's an automatic process that we take for granted and all it needs is the best building blocks for our particular combination of elements.

Six tastes

Conventional western approaches to nutrition deal with proteins, carbohydrates and calories, but in Ayurveda taste is the key issue, and there are six categories of taste that are critical to maintaining cellular health. Each taste is necessary for our immunological and spiritual functions. The essential tastes of nature, arising from the five elements, transmit vibrations that our bodies need to sustain our physical, emotional and spiritual rhythms. The vibrations help to maintain our quantum pulse. When these six tastes are absent, we suffer.

- **Sweet** is the dominant taste, produced by the water and earth elements. The sweet taste increases bodily tissue, nurtures the body and relieves hunger.

- **Sour** is formed from the earth and fire elements and helps digestion and the elimination of wastes.

- **Salty** is formed from the water and fire elements and is useful in small quantities by all types. It helps to cleanse bodily tissues and activates digestion.

- **Pungent** is formed from the elements of air and fire. It helps stimulate appetite and maintains metabolism and the balance of secretions in the body.

- **Bitter** comes from the elements of air and space, and can be used by all types in small quantities. Bitter detoxifies the blood, controls skin ailments and tones the organs.

- **Astringent** is formed from the elements of earth and air and can be used in medicinal quantities by all types. The astringent principle helps to reduce bodily secretion and constricts bodily tissue.

Let's return to an earlier theme to enlarge upon the importance of taste in Ayurveda. We are not the body we inhabit, which is a temporary assembly of particles in a particular pattern, forming a cellular structure. We are, in fact, a sustained pulse of energy, or life force and we share that characteristic with every other life form. This pulse vibrates at particular frequencies and we see and feel our world through the filter of these frequencies, which resonate throughout our cellular structure. This structure requires nourishment to maintain the vibrationary core. Well-being, balance and harmony are the result of attuning one vibration with another.

The idea of harmony and balance attracts us at an intellectual level and represents a goal that we can attain through attitudinal change, but there are fundamental practical actions and processes that sustain our vibrationary core. We resonate to our best frequency when our intake of good, natural food is balanced by our thought and actions. Food carries memory, energy and vibration from the five elements of nature into our bodies. Natural food contains the complete cycle of life within its genetic make-up and this attunes bodies to a greater cycle of life. Natural food is one of the most powerful transformers of consciousness we can engage with.

When the six tastes are absent, we lose that particular cellular memory of the five elements and we begin to lose a part of our intrinsic nature. We become dull and lose our receptivity and ability to function effectively. The presence of the six tastes in our daily food intake is critical to our welfare; they trigger responses that go deep into our psyche and which have a major impact on our awareness.

Additionally, herbs and spices have specific medicinal qualities and it is essential that we work directly with them as well as the six tastes because they enhance the tastes to trigger essential healing responses. Take notice of this: *taste is essential to healing* and often people who replace genuine nutrition with supplements are making a mistake. Much of our instinctive building and healing capability is lost when we use herbs in tablet, pill and capsule form because tablets and pills bypass the sensation of taste. Many naturally produced commercial medications are based on ingredients that originate from plants containing the quintessential medicinal pungent, bitter and astringent tastes. Unfortunately, because they are in tablet form the pungent, bitter and astringent qualities fail to trigger particular healing for specific areas of the body. As we examine the role of nutrition in Ayurveda, the concept and context of taste will be expanded upon. We'll see that conventional western diets are heavily unbalanced towards unnatural sweet and salty tastes.

What does it mean to be a 21st Century person with a particular dosha, alive in a busy world? We will examine our three case studies in situations that we've all experienced, and learn how they can work through everyday problems and decisions using Ayurvedic principles. We'll look at their lifestyles, diets, exercise regimes, choices in clothes, colour schemes, holidays and treats and make direct comparisons to understand how they feel and how we might feel in the same situation. There will be aspects of each person that you'll be able to identify with and these points of recognition are important. They will begin to reveal you to yourself and our questionnaire (Appendix A) will help you to complete the process.

It is summer in a city centre. A slim Vata type man is sitting at a café terrace eating lunch in the sun. The day is slightly breezy, but hot and dry. He's unsettled and fidgeting and seems unable to keep still. Even when it seems that he's managed to settle down and stop moving, his eyes continue darting about, and under the table a foot is constantly tapping. He's eating salad because it's healthy and non-fattening but that's creating a problem for him because he has a Vata dosha, with ether/space and air as his elements and Vata's tendency to be easily distracted. He is naturally dry because that too is a Vata tendency yet he sits in the heat with a breeze that's drying him even more. The food and surroundings contain the same elements that he is made from. He'll soon feel the effects of this interlude and become more unsettled and then he won't be able to concentrate, his behaviour will become erratic, he won't be able to make his mind up and it will all be "his fault" and he can then start to feel bad about himself all over again, another Vata tendency.

We are in a small Indian restaurant on Saturday night. This is a popular and crowded place, hot with the energy of many diners. A freckled Pitta-type woman arrives, intense and slightly annoyed, arms full of shopping, struggling to find a place for herself and her partner. She's impatient for service, flashing a fiery gaze around, tapping her table and waving the menu until she gets service. She orders a Madras curry and speaks sharply to the waiter when he tries to clarify her order. Then she calls him back to change something and acts as if it's his fault that she forgot what she wanted. Indian food could present no problems for her, but she should not be eating hot curry. She is a Pitta-type, naturally fiery and the Madras will simply spark up her inner fire and she will become unsettled and agitated, probably angry and liable to blame the waiter for everything from the weather to the state of the nation. She "deserves a treat" after the week she's had, but has pressurised herself with too much activity in the day and she's been organising her partner who she thinks "can't organise himself." Later she can't sleep and has an uncomfortable stomach all night.

A typical office scene. A large Kapha type woman sits in this tastefully cool grey working space, parked in front of her computer sipping from a bottle of cold water with some crisp-breads and cottage cheese nearby. She will soon be having a light lunch, her daily habit. She yawns a lot and seems uninterested in her work, her surroundings and the other people around her; she isn't really communicating with anyone. She doesn't seem timid and she has presence, but it's as if she's built a fence around her desk. Sadly, she thinks that no one likes her because she is overweight. She has read that water is good for flushing the system and helps weight loss, so she makes a point of drinking lots of it but what she is doing is adding to her natural tendency for fluid retention and a reluctance to become active, and she's about to eat non-fattening dairy products that fall into a taste category that Kapha-types should avoid over-doing. She's stuck in an environment with bland colours that don't help her and she is sitting passively and guaranteeing that all that starving and eating the wrong food for her body type will keep her stuck in the same rut she's been in for years.

All three of these people are eating food that isn't right for their doshas, in settings that aren't the best for them in their present state. They would be better choosing food that compliments their particular body type. They don't know it yet, but they have a foundation that hasn't changed since they were teenagers and won't ever change. One of them wants to be bigger with heavier muscles, another does a lot to remain lean and fit and the third has gradually put on weight over the years. Unless they discover more about themselves they are each simply adding to their burdens; the best thing they each can do is learn about their body type and discover how to work with it rather than against it, which is what they've all been doing for too long. When we understand our dosha and constitution we can begin to tailor our lifestyles to suit our needs, but before that can happen some work is required to discover what that dosha is.

What are the physical and emotional characteristics of these three body types?

The three examples we've just looked at are real people, clients we have worked with. Let's examine them in greater detail and for the sake of confidentiality we'll invent new names for them; let them be known as Victor, Penelope and Karen.

Client number one is Victor, a typical Vata type. He is quite tall with narrow shoulders and has thin arms and legs; he's not especially muscular but looks fit. His hair is dry and slightly wavy, dark in colour. His face is quite angular and he has a relatively thin neck for his height and size. His eyes are dark brown and deeply set and he has a tendency to dry skin. He speaks quickly and erratically with a low voice.

Victor works in the media industry and is a creative person but he's anxious and restless much of the time. He's has been bothered by stuff going on in the office but doesn't like to deal with the issues, avoiding confrontation as much as possible. His imagination and creative temperament stand him in good stead, but he and his boss know that he isn't the greatest finisher in the world. Like a lot of Vata's he has a distracted mind, often undisciplined and he finds it difficult to turn his creative visions into completed work or leisure activity.

Victor is health-conscious and keeps fit with heavy sessions on the weights, hoping to build a bulkier body. He started going to the gym with a friend with whom he's since lost contact, and he moves in a shifting circle of new friends and acquaintances. He exercises a lot but despite this is a light sleeper often getting only six hours a night despite his heavy schedule. He wants to increase his lean muscle mass through heavy weight training and is taking dietary supplements. Like many people he listens to the formulaic responses and the dogma of low fat, protein-based nutrition and he eats light salad-based meals.

Victor's flat is decorated in intense colours and textures and he goes on holiday to the Canaries, the Greek Islands (and anywhere else that's hot) with his girlfriend Charlotte, with whom he enjoys an active sex life. He and Charlotte overindulge in most things and then he becomes worried about the waste, but does nothing about it except analyse and over-analyse until he drives himself mad with it all. He socialises in clubs with loud hip-hop and dance music.

Victor has tried to chase away his anxieties with activity, but they never really go away and the chief cause of his worries is the way money seems to slip through his fingers. What bothers him most is that he never feels settled despite his good fortune and all the positive factors in his life. It is obvious that Victor is imbalanced in a number of ways. He has a good job, earns quite a lot of money and on paper does most of the things that are supposed to create joy and happiness but his moods are variable, he's anxious and unsettled and things don't seem to come easily to him.

As Linda worked with Victor she discovered that he was a typical Vata dosha. All doshas/ body types have strong characteristics and Vatas are no exception. Victor had been doing all the things he thought were "good for him", with diet, exercise and the décor of his home environment, but as Linda explained more about his dosha and its unique features, Victor began to see that the off-the-shelf standard model for healthy living that he'd been following had actually been harming him. How? Linda showed Victor what being a Vata person meant, and what kinds of food and activity would strengthen him and heal the Vata imbalances.

Vata consists of the elements of Air and Ether/space and is predominantly biased towards movement. Vata works with the nervous system to control all body movement including nutrients and waste. In the mind Vata is concerned with memory and comparison of information. It is the most common dosha found in daily life, more so over the past 100 years with the increasing levels of change and the frenetic pace that have become the norm in many societies.

Vata has particular qualities and these are: dry, light, irregular, rough, mobile, cold, quick and changeable.

How do these qualities manifest in everyday life?

Dry: A Vata type's skin will often be prone to dryness and flakiness. They may lick their fingers before touching paper, wool or other dry surfaces and may be slow to perspire compared to others They may often be thirsty. Dry humour and a tendency to irony are also Vata traits.

Light: Vata skin may be light, dull or even papery, requiring moisturising and care in all weather conditions, particularly in strong sunlight. Their body weight is usually low with a slim musculature and often with bony limbs. They may have fine hair, are often thin and can be light sleepers.

Irregular: A Vata type will have an irregular physique. They can be very tall or very short, they may have thin arms and legs and a strong torso or vice versa, a larger than average head or one that is angular, long or with a small or large chin and a nose that is prominent or small. They may have small eyes, narrow or sunken, dark brown or grey in colour, and irregular teeth. They may suffer from delicate appetites, frequent constipation or have irregular bowel movements and flatulence.

Rough: Unevenness of responses, excessive contrasts and a lack of free flow and smoothness in speech and actions all manifest as roughness with Vata types. Their speech may be lacking in modulation, they may "feel rough" and show visible signs of wear and tear when fatigued. They may develop rough skin and complexions, especially when older. They may have a "rough idea" of something and be "rough and ready" or unkempt and untidy regardless of what they wear. Roughness can be manifested through coarseness or a lack of softness in everything from behaviour to the texture of skin, clothes and habitat.

Mobile: Vata types never stop moving physically or mentally and this is often manifested as restlessness. This both strengthens and weakens their natural creativity, because the ability to move and shift can often lead to creative impulses but it can also prevent tasks being completed. They have strong imaginations and are likely to be artistic or in the creative professions. They often express themselves through sport and are sexually active. Mobility is also manifested as anxiety, fearfulness, questioning and theorising and an ability to spend money easily. When balanced, Vata types achieve many things and when unbalanced they appear disconnected from themselves.

Cold: Seasonal change affects Vata types more than others. They feel the cold easily and are susceptible to drafts, yet under the right circumstances and with preparation they cope with winter weather, provided that they wear suitable fleecy clothing. (If they turn up the heating to compensate for the cold they soon dry out and develop dry roughened skin.) Vata types can also be emotionally cold, finding it difficult to sustain close relationships.

Quick: Vata types think, move, speak and act quickly. They spend quickly, often on the wrong things; they make speedy decisions and are likely to reverse them just as quickly. They fall quickly into agitated states and can be moved quickly out of them, provided awareness is developed. Vata types remember things quickly and forget them quickly.

Changeable: Everything about Vata types is changeable. We have already mentioned seasonal change, but change has a more profound effect on them more than other doshas because it compounds their inherent changeability. They veer from enthusiasm and intensity to despondency and anxiety, from happiness to joy, from physical balance to unco-ordinated chaos and they do all of this quickly; their emotionl states can change with the speed of a cloud passing across the sun. A Vata type's thought patterns can inspire themselves and all around them, or drive everyone to distraction. Being a Vata type can involve considerable confusion and discomfort when unbalanced. They are creative and welcome new experiences but do not like routine. However, they NEED routine to stabilise their mental patterns and moods. Vata types can easily become out of balance mentally, emotionally and physically, and can be indecisive and often fearful in their life environment.

All of these qualities increase with age in Vata types.

In our bodies Vata is responsible for: thinking, respiration, circulation and digestive movement. All of these qualities are necessary in all body types and we wouldn't function without the Vata qualities of movement, nor would we function without the space through which fluids, food and air can pass. These qualities are simply more evident in a Vata type and they become excessive when Vata become imbalanced.

Vata types are better suited to structured exercise classes such as aerobics or circuit training, swimming, walking, properly organised jogging, mountain activity, Yoga and Tai Chi and some Martial Arts activities, and much less suited to heavy weight-based exercise regimes.

Balanced Vata types are energetic and inspirational, adapt to situations, and are lively, creative and good communicators.

Unbalanced Vata types worry; they are agitated, restless and full of anxiety. They are inconsistent and often suffer from insomnia. They can be gassy, bloated and constipated.

A typical Vata stress response is "What did I do wrong?" reminding us of a child needing Mummy or Daddy to get them out of a fix. Vatas assume responsibility for errors and avoid confrontation.

A Vata type can be summarised as having a variable and changeable character.

Victor went through a detailed analysis with Linda and soon saw the kinds of physical attributes and patterns in his behaviour that confirmed him as a Vata body type. When a Vata person like Victor becomes out of balance, all of the functions listed become impaired and every quality becomes exaggerated, as they do with all out of balance doshas. The worry and anxiety that he suffered were tendencies that a Vata person is always prone to. His choice of holiday destinations didn't really suit him because Vata types are already dry and he kept on choosing very hot dry places to go to. Trying to achieve muscular bulk through heavy weight training was doubly wrong for him, because his body type wouldn't develop to the levels of the bodybuilders in the magazines, and salads and light food were all wrong for someone who is already light and full of air and who was putting his body through such rigours.

Victor learned that he could regain balance through correct nutrition and by changing his routines for exercise, work, sleep and his domestic life, and he also learned that his emotional life and the practical daily acts of living were interwoven. Although change had always unsettled him he knew it would always occur because change is a fact of life, so he needed to be aware of what was going on both outside and inside himself and learn not to get unconsciously caught up with worrying about it. Easily said, but Linda described how visualisation techniques and the development of his senses would strengthen his ability to focus on nurturing experiences.

For Victor the changes would mean that he shouldn't eat and do things that increased any of the characteristics that he already had, because that would aggravate the natural tendencies of air and space that were already quite excessive. Every aspect of Victor's lifestyle would come under scrutiny, but to start with Linda showed him how attention to the six tastes would make a dramatic difference to his well-being and especially to the three tastes most suited to his Vata dosha. Vata types consist of the pungent, bitter and astringent tastes. Victor should have been balancing them with the three elements of earth, water and fire found in the sweet, sour and salty tastes.

With Linda's guidance he began to see how to go about creating large and small changes to his life.

Client number two is Penelope. She is a typical Pitta type, a vivacious lively woman with intense blue eyes and a direct gaze, well-defined cheekbones and jaw line, a petite nose and a positive open smile. Her dark red hair is fine but lustrous and beautifully groomed. She has a lean, healthy and compact physique with well-toned muscles.

Penelope is a teacher and because of her obvious organisational gifts and qualities of leadership she has progressed quickly from her initial training to being a relatively young Deputy Head in an inner city school that faces challenges. Many of the staff are tired and unmotivated, unhappy with policies that the new Headmaster wants to implement and she is frustrated by their combination of apathy and resistance. She sees what needs to be done, wants to move things forward as quickly as possible and becomes angry at their unwillingness to see her point of view. She has had a number of angry confrontations with key staff and has reacted badly each time.

As a schoolgirl she was athletic and competitive and still remains active with badminton and intense aerobic workouts. She enjoys clubbing and dancing till the early hours whenever she can. Whether she's keeping fit or clubbing Penelope stays hydrated with lots of citrus drinks. She's conscious of her fitness and wants to step up the aerobic workouts, thinking she might take up "boxercise" with friends who say how great it is for getting rid of aggression.

Penelope has a fiery and demanding long-term relationship. Her boyfriend often goes away with his friends on mountain climbing trips and that leads to arguments and accusations of divided loyalties since she finds some of his friends egotistical and brash. They nevertheless have an intense and passionate relationship, with plenty of socialising and several trips per year, using her school holiday time to visit hot exotic places such as Morocco, Andalusia and the like. When they go away she always organises a busy schedule of places to visit, cramming lots of value into each trip. However, her boyfriend's lackadaisical attitude often disrupts her plans, leading to arguments.

She is fond of eating out and likes spicy Tapas and Indian food. At school cheese and pickles are one of her favourite lunchtime choices, with salsa dips. Sometimes she suffers from indigestion and tries to ease it with branded products or yoghurt which, she believes, has soothing qualities. She drinks wine with every meal and is a good cook specialising in spicy Mediterranean dishes, using her holiday experiences to expand her repertoire. She always has yoghurt for breakfast.

Penelope has lived with her boyfriend for 7 years in a small house filled with rich wall hangings and textiles from their trips to North Africa. She wears strong, dramatic colours most of the time and has a lot of easy-care synthetic and mixed fabrics in her wardrobe, many of them intended for outdoor activities, that also make a teacher's busy life easier to manage.

Linda worked with Penelope and it didn't take much to figure out that she was a real Pitta dosha with strong qualities of drive and determination, and an intense desire to change things. Her professional and personal life was almost overpoweringly intense, with competitive activities in the gym compounding the pressure she put herself under. Her choice of colours and fabrics in clothing inflamed her Pitta tendencies, as did the décor of her home, and though she was a strong and independent woman, she didn't do anything to nurture herself. She had been throwing petrol on her Pitta fire for a long time and needed cooling down with a new regime. Linda shone some light on Penelope's natural Pitta qualities and it became clear that food, activities and environmental factors were all in need of change.

Pitta consists of the elements of Fire and Water and is predominantly biased towards transformation. Fire and water govern the body's balance of chemical and transforming energies, including the digestion of both food and thought. In the mind Pitta processes new data and draws conclusions.

Pitta has particular qualities and these are: light, hot, intense, medium, sharp, penetrating, pungent, and acidic.

How do these qualities manifest in everyday life?

Light: Digestion, the processing of bulk and waste and activation of the body's natural cleansing activities are served by this Pitta quality, which helps create the balanced Pitta traits of freshness and alertness. In an unbalanced state this can lead to ungroundendess. Pitta types suffer sore eyes when in very bright light and will usually be seen with sunglasses a lot of the time, but they also need enough good quality daylight to maintain a positive emotional outlook.

Hot: Pitta types may be physically hot and prone to perspiration, finding hot summer days difficult to cope with and tending to sunburn. Despite this they have lustrous skin and good complexions when in balance. Unfortunately Pitta types are also prone to hot flushes and rashes when unbalanced. They are passionate with hot tempers and are quick to become involved in heated exchanges with others. When balanced this passion makes them good leaders. Heat is an essential component of digestion and most transformative processes but because Pitta types have this natural heat, hot spicy food can aggravate them. Unbalanced Pitta heat can lead to inflammation, anger and hate.

Intense: Pitta types are often keen, intelligent, alert and highly focussed and make good leaders, teachers and advocates. They have intense relationships with equal measures of humour and argument. Their passions lead them to great lengths in support, defence or promotion of what matters to them. They have intense arguments and won't concede easily. Intensity can be both positive and negative and Pitta types can be intensely roused and capable of moving mountains or intensely shut down, inactive and depressed. They feel the highs and lows of emotions, circumstances and events deeply.

Medium: This quality epitomises the essence of a Pitta's balanced attributes. A balanced Pitta type can see both sides of a story; they eat well, neither gorging nor starving; they plan their days and work through an agenda without Vata airiness or Kapha lethargy; and they are in control of their lives. When unbalanced this instinct to control becomes excessive and then Pitta types become overpowering and dominating. They have balanced physiques, regardless of height, with well-proportioned limbs necks and torsos, good musculature and a capacity for endurance-based exercise. They have balanced facial features and clear strong voices. Pitta hair can be fine and soft, fair or reddish in colour, prone to premature greying but often lustrous and of good quality.

Sharp: Pitta types have can have clear-cut features, such as a pointed chin or nose. They can be intelligent and have quick minds, sharp humour, grasp ideas easily and are articulate. Pitta types are "on the ball"; they work quickly and act decisively, especially under duress and a Pitta type is likely to be the one who takes charge in an emergency. Their conversation can be sharp and prickly in tone even when not aroused and they can be irritable, jealous or aggressive. When unwell they can experience sharp pain wherever their sickness is located and this kind of pain is useful when diagnosing Pitta imbalances in any dosha.

Penetrating: Pitta types will have a penetrating gaze and the ability to get behind the smoke screens that many people put around themselves. They can see through hidden agendas but can also be judgemental in their comments. They are discriminating, able to organise ideas, arguments and other people, are quick learners and have good insight and memory. This quality is also evident in less dramatic ways; Pitta's ability to penetrate often requires persistence, the capacity to ask searching questions and a willingness to dig behind the surface of appearances.

Pungent: This hottest and driest quality creates thirst and discomfort in Pitta types who are likely to need water in the middle of the night, and along with their natural heat will seek out cold spots under the bedclothes. Pungency can be overpowering and forceful; in food the pungent tastes are used sparingly because of their strength, and an unbalanced Pitta type can be "over the top" exhibiting overbearing behaviour, often accompanied by pungent body odour. Balanced Pitta pungency has that edgy quality that snaps things into focus.

Acidic: Pitta qualities are specifically connected to digestive fire and the transformative processes that require acid as a key ingredient. Balance is critical however and unbalanced Pitta states create corrosive levels of acidity leading to stomach pain, ulcers, critical attitudes, often involving biting and cutting remarks. Acidity is essential for transformation but damaging when present in excess.

These qualities are manifested in a Pitta's behaviour, conversation, looks, sleep patterns, tendency to perspire easily, reaction to hot food and weather.

In our bodies Pitta is responsible for mental discrimination, visual perception, body temperature, skin and complexion, digestion. All of these qualities are found in all body types and are essential for normal life. We couldn't function without the Pitta ability to transform and digest food, ideas and our perception. They are simply more obvious in Pitta types and become exaggerated when Pittas become unbalanced.

Pitta body types are usually of medium build with average proportions of legs and arms and even fingers and toes, with good musculature. They often have fine hair that may be prematurely grey. They perspire easily, often with a keen odour, are passionate and have average levels of sleep. A Pitta type will be prone to hot temper and strong digestion.

Pitta types have sharp intellects and are direct and to the point; they prefer routine, have the courage of their conviction and make good teachers and leaders. They are good with money but like luxuries. They will be driven emotionally, physically and mentally.

A Pitta type can be summarised as being vigorous and fiery.

Pitta types are better suited to relaxation activities such as Yoga, Tai Chi or Qi Gong, walking, swimming, meditation practise, moderate weight-based activities and natural environments. They are much less suited to aggressive, competitive games.

Balanced Pitta types make good decisions, are good leaders, are warm, bright and intelligent and have good digestion.

Unbalanced Pitta types are prone to anger, irritability and can be critical and judgemental. They can have skin problems and burning heated complaints.

A typical Pitta stress response is "What did you do wrong?"

Linda worked through a detailed analysis of Penelope's dosha qualities and her well-balanced physique and emotional disposition confirmed her dosha. It didn't take long for Penelope's anger to show itself when she talked about her frustrations. Pitta types prefer routine and organisation. For much of the time things were out of control and this aggravated Penelope's Pitta character.

Penelope had taken herself into a position of confrontation at work because she believed passionately in what was required. She had prided herself on the ability to organise and cope with a demanding workload, but the attitude of her staff was creating problems. She'd never felt stressed before but now it was becoming a problem. However, things were never boring and she still enjoyed a good argument. As soon as she got in her car to go home it was all forgotten with loud rock music blasting out of the stereo.

She rationalised that people would soon realise she was right all along. The rows with her boyfriend were only because he couldn't see the truth in what she was saying—he was impossible at times. Poor digestion and some skin problems had been bothering her but she had put that down to stress, the situation in school and the weather. She suffered from hot sweats at night and heavy perspiration when tense or under stress. All her problems were actually a manifestation of her imbalanced Pitta state.

Penelope's life had in fact become a hothouse of tensions at work and at home, fuelled by power colours, hot food and hot weather in the holiday breaks. When a Pitta type's natural qualities of organisation and leadership become imbalanced for any reason, this turns into anger and exasperation very easily. It was vital that she learned to bring some peace into her life and reduce the damaging levels of tension she was exposed to by re-examining her diet, activities and leisure pursuits and the way she dealt with workplace tensions. She was badly in need of calming, meditative experiences in her life and of the cooling influences that all Pitta types need to counteract their natural heat and these experiences were what Linda introduced her to, with earth, air and space being key elements.

Like Victor, Penelope did not need to increase any of the characteristics that she already had; she was already out of balance. She needed to pay attention to her whole way of living, beginning with attention to the six tastes that would make the same dramatic difference to Penelope's wellbeing as they would to Victor and Karen. Pitta types consist of the sour, salty and pungent tastes and Penelope should have been balancing them with the three elements of earth, air and space found in the sweet, astringent and bitter tastes.

Large and small changes were to be a part of her life too.

Client number three is Karen. She has an open face with beautiful big brown eyes, thick brown hair and a wide, full smile accentuated by full lips. Her face is strong but not bony. She has always had a good figure with shapely legs and hips but she's put weight on and become more "well-covered" than she wants to be. Her voice is quite low and her speech measured.

She has worked for the same company for 15 years and is a senior programmer and administrator in IT systems. She is one of the cornerstones of the company but is unhappy with recent changes to company policy and structure and to the new working patterns recently brought in. Although she's responsible for managing change and should have been re-structuring the work within her area of responsibility she finds it very difficult to energise herself into action with her staff and needs a lot of encouragement from her line manager even to get to the point of reviewing her staff's workloads.

When younger she was an active walker and swimmer, with life-saving medals to her credit but she had stopped these activities some time ago. She has been meeting her friend at the sports centre once a week for yoga class for the past 5 years and they sometimes go out for country walks together. They also go away together on holiday every summer and winter for away-breaks in nice hotels, often close to a beach. She sleeps very heavily and is happy to stay in with a good book at weekends.

Karen has read every diet book under the sun (and tried most of them) but her weight only increases despite low-fat meals and all the other fads. She actually eats quite small meals and drinks lots of fluid. She loves yoghurt and cheese, but is careful how much she eats, and has plenty of fruit juice and water throughout the day. Her speciality at home is light pasta and rice meals with tomatoes and courgettes accompanied by mild sauces, or couscous and other Mediterranean dishes with yoghurt accompaniments, and hummus, often with wholemeal bread and crackers. Generally, Karen thinks that she takes care of her calories. When she eats out she likes Chinese food, especially sweet and sour flavours. At home she likes the odd box of chocolates with her evening television, but not every night. However she also sneaks in a biscuit or two and a packet of crisps. These are comfort foods. She was divorced six years ago after six years of marriage to a man with whom she enjoyed an easy and relaxed sexual relationship; at this point there is no one else on the horizon. She sees her nieces and nephews most weeks and has the younger ones for overnight stays as often as they want to come. Family parties are high on her agenda.

Karen has lived in the same house for 12 years and before that was in the same neighbourhood for over 10 years, where she lived with her family. The house is decorated in a motley collection of un-coordinated colours and textures that actually match Karen's wardrobe of bright, extravagant clothing that she's had for years. She keeps thinking she might move to a newer property but isn't really keen on the upheaval of moving house, what with the changes at work to deal with as well. She knows she is reluctant to make the necessary changes in her working life but she realises that this kind of thing happens from time to time and usually blows over, so she keeps her own counsel until the problem goes away.

Karen was honest when responding to Linda's analysis of her dosha and it was very obvious how typical she was of the Kapha type. Her physique and looks were distinctly Kapha; open, clear-eyed, solid and strong with a tendency to heaviness that occurs with imbalance. The resistance to change in her professional life, combined with a long-standing routine of holidays and weekend activities indicated a tendency towards lethargy that is also a Kapha trait. She was stuck in a rut of her own making, compounded by her apparent good intentions with food and drink and her sense of décor and her wardrobe. Rather than place herself in the kind of stimulating situations and environments that Kapha types could benefit from she existed in a kind of wall-to-wall blandness. Linda opened her up to new, spicier opportunities.

Kapha consists of the elements of Earth and Water and is predominantly biased towards stability. Kapha calmness governs structure, bodily stability and lubrication and cell structure. In the mind Kapha provides stability and the ability to grasp single thoughts.

Kapha has particular qualities and these are:

Heavy: Kapha has substance. Kapha types have physical and emotional weight and the capacity to build and increase substance as a central aspect of the whole process of nutrition. Kapha types can have a serious approach to many issues, a willingness to embrace complexity and a "heaviness" and depth that is reassuring to those around them. When unbalanced this can lead to excessive physical weight, lethargy, even laziness and heavy handedness. They can become dull, often as a protective measure, since dulling the senses shields them from pain and difficulty; they feel burdened and often bored.

Solid: Balanced Kapha types are enduring characters with reliable natures, "salt of the earth" individuals around whom communities grow and flourish. They have sound judgement and sturdy self-belief. They are the strongest of the body types, with powerful core physiques, thick limbs and broad torsos, rounded features and quite large eyes and mouth, thick hair and thick skin that can be pale and cool. They are capable of hard physical effort. When unbalanced this solidity turns to stubbornness, a "lack of give and take" and a one-track narrow-mindedness.

Stable: Kapha types are calm steady and considerate individuals, patient, stable and slow to anger. There is an air of security around them. When balanced they have reliable, unchanging personalities and possess a steady consistency around which other people are comfortable. They do not get agitated and make good listeners, the kind of people we can go to with a problem. When unbalanced they become inflexible and resistant to change and this can lead to possessive and obsessive behaviour.

Cold: Kapha types are often physically or emotionally cool. They are affected by cool weather and withdraw into hibernation when possible. This coolness can help them when under pressure. When unbalanced, however, coolness becomes emotional detachment, denial and withdrawal. Often an appearance of aloofness masks insecurity and a loss of that essential Kapha sense of self.

Smooth: In a positive balanced state this quality brings assuredness, evenness and grace. Kapha types can be excellent dancers, exhibiting effortless movement. Kapha skin is smooth and free from blemishes and their actions and speech are slow and rhythmic. When unbalanced these qualities lead to slickness and a "smooth talking" way of dealing with issues, a slippery evasiveness and a tendency to hide feelings that can lead to passive aggressive behaviour that masks an unwillingness to co-operate.

Slow: Kapha types are deliberate and measured and tend to be slow to learn something new but even slower to forget. They are visibly unhurried and a Kapha type's slow methodical nature allows them to resist pressure, avoiding wrong decisions and action. They excel in logical analysis and take time in reaching conclusions which are correspondingly well-founded. When unbalanced this quality becomes excessive and they almost grind to a halt, such is their slowness, even to the point of sluggishness in any activity. They need long hours of sleep.

Structured: Balanced Kapha types are the building block of families, societies and businesses. They have the most solid constitutions of all the doshas. They are organised, ordered, reliable and stable at a deep personal level. They can build structure and organisation into their personal and professional lives and help others to move to solid ground. When unbalanced they become rigid and inflexible, unable to change direction or the basis of their thinking.

These qualities become manifested in a Kapha's behaviour and approach to most aspects of life, in their salt of the earth character, their unwillingness to confront difficulty, their manner of speech and thought, their tendency to gain weight easily and their unwillingness to undertake major change.

Kapha is responsible for Nurturing the nervous system, lubricating joints and the digestive tract, regulating water and regulating fat. All body types require these Kapha functions to operate properly. The Kapha qualities of fluidity enable us to move with ease internally and in the external physical world. They are simply more evident in a Kapha type and become problematical when a Kapha is unbalanced.

Kapha body types are usually of heavier build with thick, full and often oily hair, strong solid legs, thick arms and shoulders. They gain weight easily and lose it with difficulty, sleep deeply and soundly and are slow to action.

Kapha types are easy-going, patient and prefer routine. They are usually devoted caregivers and are good with money and savings. A Kapha type is someone who is solid in structure, easily puts on weight and really dislikes any change.

A Kapha type can be summarised as being grounded and earthy.

Kapha types are better suited to heavy or explosive activity such as weightlifting, sprinting or any intense workout and are physically strong. They make good dancers, being light on their feet despite their heavier build.

Balanced Kapha types are steady, consistent, strong and supportive.

Unbalanced Kapha types are prone to hoarding and can be lethargic, overweight, needy and lazy.

A typical Kapha stress response is "I don't want to know."

With Linda's guidance Karen was quick to see what a classic Kapha body type she was in most respects, from her physique and behaviour to her emotional state, which had become lethargic and resistant to new experiences. When younger her Kapha strength and reliability had enabled her to weather most storms, whether personal or professional, but at some point she had shut herself down. As a typically out of balance Kapha, Karen had withdrawn into herself and settled for the same old everything and it was only the forced changes at work that might have pushed her into action, but she was even resisting these potentially liberating circumstances.

The steady routine in her life and work had become too comfortable and like many Kaphas, when change reared its head she, who had been a great planner and organiser for the company in her early days, became quiet and fearful. She had shut down at work just as she had done in her domestic life and had spent years in a rut becoming complacent and apathetic.

She had avoided the spicy foods and lively environments that would have been great for balancing her natural Kapha tendency to shut down, and Linda began to work with her to develop a new plan for shifting her life. Correct nutrition for her Kapha dosha would begin help her achieve her natural weight which she would be happier with, encouraging more physical activity, a hunger for new situations, challenge and excitement and renewed vigour.

Karen did not need to increase any of the characteristics that she already had; she was out of balance. She was already full of Kapha sweetness and liked sour tastes but ate food that added to that sweetness, sourness and saltiness without realising what she was doing. The fluids she drank in quite large quantities were also not helping her Kapha body type. Like Victor and Penelope, Karen needed to pay attention to her whole way of living beginning with the six tastes. Kapha types consist of the sweet, sour and salty tastes and Karen should have been balancing them with the three elements of ether/space, air and fire found in the pungent, astringent and bitter tastes.

Exciting changes were in store for Karen.

For all doshas

It is important to realise that the five elements of nature, the building blocks of all life are within each dosha and that it is simply the differing balances between these elements that create the individual doshas. These same elements are within our food in the form of the six tastes. Appendix A contains a questionnaire that will help you to determine your own dosha. Remember that we are all combinations of each of the three main doshas and that you are likely to consist of one main dosha followed closely by a secondary dosha. We will discuss ways of dealing with your combination dosha in Chapter 7. For now we suggest that you complete the questionnaire so that the journey that our three case studies take becomes more relevant to you. Instructions for completing the questionnaire are included in Appendix A. Appendix B contains a chart of the elements and Appendix C a chart of the six tastes. These will help you to select your food types and locate them into your Ayurvedic profile as you work through the experiences of our three subjects.

This information has been built up over thousands of years of practical experience. It is no surprise that it can work for each of our three case studies, even though they are all different body types. One of the many benefits to anyone who follows Ayurvedic practises is the knowledge that we can take control of so much of our lives through very simple daily acts that include preparing and cooking delicious food, and through attention to our environment and the activities we undertake. Care and attention to all other aspects of living transform our human experience and here too Ayurveda guides us through the choices we make about the physical and spiritual factors in our lives. For now we will leave you to review the opportunities created by Ayurveda's six tastes in your life plan. In Chapter 3 we look in greater depth at the implications of tastes on our client's health.

Chapter 2

Quantum Theory
and the
Five Elements

There is an oft-quoted saying that "we are all one" and it is true in a physical as well as a spiritual sense. We truly are interconnected at the deepest level. What we do to ourselves we do to all other life forms and to our planet. Our thoughts and intentions have massive potential energy and the capacity to create physical outcomes that affect our health, all aspects of our lives and much more. We know people who "carry the weight of the world on their shoulders" and others who "bounce for joy," and we can all see the socio-economic consequences of low expectations and low self-esteem in communities and large chunks of our society. A buoyant outlook and sense of optimism help to create circumstances that lead to happiness and satisfaction with life and, conversely, negative expectations too often become a self-fulfilling recipe for depression and unhappiness. We are what we think and we affect everything around us through our thoughts and attitudes. How does this happen?

Current thinking in the 20th and 21st Century in the realms of physics and mathematics offers explanations for knowledge and beliefs that have existed for over 5000 years. Philosophers and most of the major world religions tell us that we are all connected and that what we do to one we do to all. This belief has formed the core of spiritual practise across different cultures. However the conviction that we are all one and connected at a deep level has, over time, become submerged. Nowadays, for many, the concept of interdependent life, of connections between living things hardly extends to families, neighbours and fellow countrymen, let alone life outside the immediate daily realm. It has most certainly faded at the level of international interests. If our leaders, and hence ourselves, truly believed in oneness and unity, we would not see wars and famine; we would not see "fellow believers" from similar faiths committing outrages against one another in the name of God, or nationalism, or any other reason; we wouldn't see excessive concern with national interests and barely disguised colonialism from the richest nations. A sense of spiritual and physical connection is now assumed by most to be of an ethereal nature, one that has no concrete explanation at the level of physical reality but, rather one which formed a kind of paternalistic code by which the highest form of life—humanity—could "manage" and care for other forms of life.

The growth of industrial and post-industrial society and commerce has led most of the Western world and now large portions of the Eastern world away from the faith that kept this belief in spiritual and physical connection alive in a living practical sense. "We are all one" is now to most people a concept more relating to markets and economies; it has been left to the environmentalists to lead the most recent debates concerning the inter-relatedness of life on our planet.

It is obvious that we share our world with other species and life forms, but how are we connected? What are the implications of any connection, if proven in the light of 21st Century scientific knowledge? In order to answer that question we will look at some of the certainties that existed in the minds of scientists from the tradition of Classical Physics which held sway until the 1900's and which still help to explain a "common sense" view of the universe. We will look at the challenges to that orthodoxy, initiated by Einstein and developed by other leading figures since that have turned those notions upside down. Physicists' viewpoints regarding the workings of our universe have changed significantly, creating theories that have withstood rigorous mathematical testing and experimental data that correlates precisely with these theories, and appearing to solve many anomalies that classical physics could not explain. Through developments in technology scientists have been able to examine the universe at deeper microscopic levels than ever before revealing characteristics and behaviour between microscopic components unforeseen in classical physics. These observations reveal the true relationship between what had previously been seen as separate, independent forms and structures.

Early Views of Physics

A Newtonian view of physics provides the classical "common sense" view of the universe. It was a mathematical framework that can still explain the everyday experience of being alive and it involved four assumptions about the fabric of reality known as reality, locality, causality and continuity. We can understand these assumptions intuitively.

Reality is the assumption that the world is real; things are things and exist independently whether we observe them or not and space and time are absolute and fixed. **Locality** is the assumption that objects can only be influenced by direct contact and not by any actions conducted at distance. **Causality** is the assumption that time is one-directional, the basis for the fixed nature of cause and effect sequences. Events only ever occur in a particular sequence. **Continuity** assumes that space and time are smooth and that sequence governs actions with no sudden leaps in natural progressions.

These assumptions governed the view of a sequential and logical universe that we could understand intuitively and that corresponded to the everyday experience of reality. Even 20th century understanding of these assumptions got people across oceans and continents, harnessed various forms of energy, informed medical progress and got man to the moon. The universe was a stable place consisting of predictable units following predictable courses.

The ancient Greeks had worked out that the universe was built up from ingredients that were the smallest building blocks of existence and we get the word "atom" from them. They believed that atoms in varying concentrations made up everything in the material world and that belief persisted more or less intact into the 20th Century. Newton's four assumptions (reality, locality, causality and continuity) described formal structures and processes that were founded upon this principle. However, by the 1930's Einstein had developed his two Theories of Relativity that completely revised the scientific establishment's views on the relationship between mass, energy, space and time. Einstein's theories changed the way science perceives the grand, universal themes.

Since then **Quantum Mechanics** has emerged as a conceptual framework for understanding the microscopic properties of the universe. Quantum Mechanics has demonstrated that at the microscopic scale the universe is absolutely chaotic and unpredictable. Classical Newtonian divisions between energy and matter hardly exist. In fact energy can become matter and vice versa. Physicists have learned that nothing is what it seems and that at the deepest microscopic level all existence, all life forms are in a fundamental state of flux. Discoveries and theoretical models, since proven under experimental conditions, completely changed the notion of permanence and solidity. The world is definitely not what it seems. The apparent stability of the classical physicist's view of the world could never be the same again once powerful technologies allowed microscopic study at levels previously unattainable. All that had been defined previously as objectively real was in a state of continual change at the microscopic level. Things were held together not by absolute construction in space and time, but by a continual dance of particles and waves.

We now know that atoms are not the smallest particles but that they consist of a nucleus, containing protons and neutrons surrounded by a cluster of orbiting electrons. Protons and neutrons consist of smaller particles called quarks. Everything in the terrestrial world and beyond consists of electrons, up-quarks and down-quarks. Experimental evidence exists of a fourth particle called a neutrino, a much less concrete kind of particle, one that travels through matter without hindrance. Neutrinos can travel through trillions of miles of lead without impedance and billions of neutrinos ejected by the sun pass through space and through our bodies all the time.

Four fundamental forces are at work: the gravitational force (gravity), the electromagnetic force, the prosaically named weak force, and the strong force. In various ways these forces keep particles together. Gravity keeps our feet on the ground and our planet in orbit. Gravity also allows us to measure mass, which is the amount of gravitational force an object can exert and receive. The electromagnetic force drives our world—light, machinery, telephones—everything that we live and work with. At one end of the scale it creates thunder and lightning and at the other it permeates to the sub-atomic level and creates the microscopic surges of electricity within our nervous system that allow us to feel, touch and sense our world. The strong and the weak forces were discovered only recently and they operate at the sub-atomic level as nuclear forces. The strong force glues quarks together inside protons and neutrons and within the atomic nuclei, and the weak force is responsible for the radioactive decay of substances. There is a huge spread in the relative strength of these forces, with the electromagnetic being far and away the strongest by a factor of billions. Were it not balanced by the fact that things have an equal amount of positive and negative charges, which cancel each other out, then the electromagnetic force would overwhelm gravity. Although gravity is a much weaker force it is constant and without any counter forces, so that more mass means a stronger gravitational force. The strong and weak forces keep all particles in particular arrangements and balance out opposing gravitational or electromagnetic forces at the tiny sub-atomic scale. Atomic nuclei would disintegrate without these forces gluing them together. This mixture of elements exists at the scale of the greatest star and at the scale of a single cell from a living creature.

Quantum Mechanics

In 1905 Einstein solved one of the problems relating to the photoelectric properties of light. His work laid the foundation for others to establish that the whole fabric of reality is subject to change and influence from the act of observation. Quantum mechanics developed a sound theoretical base for the belief that observation and creation are interrelated and that consciousness creates reality.

The background to this discovery lay in studies of the photoelectric properties of light, which can cause the release of electrons from the surface of certain metals as a result of the transfer of energy. Einstein established that light should be thought of as a stream of particles—photons—and that each photon had sufficient energy to cause change, hence electrons being knocked from the metal. Other work also showed that light has wave characteristics. Particles, or electrons are separate objects in microscopic space that are relatively hard. Under experimental conditions, when hurled at each other with great force they can be seen to destroy each other, releasing massive amounts of energy. In this context, light, seen as a stream of particles, has the capacity to change that which it falls upon. The wave characteristics of light are like soft undulations in water. They are not localised but spread out, and they are soft in that they can interact without destroying each other. Depending on how you measure it light behaves with particle characteristics, emitting photons that can affect what they come into contact with and it also behaves with all the characteristics of a wave, creating patterns, peaks and troughs in exactly the way that waves in water behave, with interference patterns and cross wave effects. Other experimentation proved that electrons (matter) behave with the same dual characteristics, having particle and wave properties, further undermining old certainties regarding permanence and stability within the microscopic universe. None of these discoveries tallied with a common sense view of the world, but have been, nevertheless, conclusively proven over the past 80 years.

Electrons and all other components of the universe cannot be located accurately in time and space, since the act of observing them, of "shining a light on them," disturbs them and causes a reaction. The act of pinpointing the location of these most microscopic of elements has been likened to trying to locate a submerged rock accurately from the wave patterns in the surrounding sea. Disturbances to the general trend of waves tell us that the rock is there somewhere but not with pinpoint accuracy. We view a pattern and make predictions based on where we predict or suppose that rock to be. Scientists now use this wave analogy to describe the world. Things are never what they seem and are never exactly where we think they are. They can in fact be in several places at once. All microscopic components are subject to variables governed by probability in the way that larger waves in the sea are likely to appear in certain places and not others. We learn that particles can vanish, cancelled out by equal opposing forces just as a trough can absorb a wave. The matter that we see as solid objects is subject at the microscopic level to the same fluctuations and electromagnetic pulse and the same laws of probability as a wave in the ocean.

Within all this detail is the realisation that all of these states of being, the balance of forces and the "gluing" together of particles is impermanent and subject to change and fluctuation from moment to moment and subject to influence from the act of observation itself! Creation—of mass, of solidity, of energy—is in a constant state of movement. The neutrons, protons and electrons that make up everything we see are in a continual state of agitation. Quantum mechanics tells us that all possibilities exist at any given moment in our universe. All particles carry the same potential for energy. Differences in frequencies and wavelengths between clusters of particles create our perception of the "solid world" and we learn that probability is a key factor in determining where a particle shows itself.

We are now forced to the conclusion that the physical world is not fixed but changes according to how we observe it. **Reality**, one of Newton's four assumptions, is no longer absolute. The things we observe may appear real intuitively, but at deep microscopic levels they are all in a state of flux. **Nonlocality** now defines the condition in which objects that are apparently separate are actually connected through space-time. **Causality** no longer stands up as an assumption because we now know from the work of Einstein and others that sequences of events dependon the perspectives of the observers. Anomalies are now seen to exist in space and time, so the assumption of **continuity** fades.

A great deal of work over the past 80 years since Einstein's breakthrough theories, has consolidated scientific thinking on quantum mechanics and the changed perception of the relationship between appearances and microscopic reality. **String theory** is the most recent development. Building upon quantum mechanics, the central principle of string theory is that everything at the most microscopic level consists of combinations of vibrating strands. The observed particles that we see are reflections of the way that strings can vibrate. Particles are really combinations of vibrating filaments that resonate at particular frequencies. The mass and force of a particle, and hence the objects in a "visible world," are determined by the patterns of oscillation of the strings. We are familiar with the way that a vibrating guitar string will produce a note and that this note can vary according to the pitch of the oscillation. String theory sees this relationship occurring at the most sub-microscopic scale within all matter and forces. These vibrations unify the incredible range and spread of particle properties into cohesive form.

For all of this body of research, theoretical predictions, based on mathematical models, have withstood repeated experimentation. The classical common sense view of the universe helps to understand everyday "reality" but if the universe behaves according to the theories, which seems to be the case, a much grander reality exists beyond the special limited perspective that held sway until now. What is interesting is the movement within the scientific community towards a belief in unity between all that exists at the Quantum level. A lot of information exists, much of it highly specialised and mind-bogglingly difficult to understand, on the development of Quantum theory and the revised viewpoint the scientific community takes of the universe and its working. The reader should look to many other excellent sources for further detailed information.

These facts and theories help scientists and the lay person to understand the mechanics of existence. They do not explain the profundity of human experience or the human capacity for joy and sorrow nor the range between these polarities. Many people balk at the thought that our emotional life is simply the product of chemical reactions in the brain caused by the "dance" of particles, molecules, atoms and their vibrating strings of energy. Science does not have all the answers and many believe that our capacity to experience thoughts and emotions, to make choices and live in consequence of these choices is where the goal and the mystery of life reside. What string theory and quantum mechanics confirm beyond doubt is that we do have control over the lives that we create. We have the ability to work with and to affect our vibratory frequencies. We are not pre-determined to be miserable, sick or emotionally damaged and we can raise our levels of vibration to create and enhance the quality of life. We can work directly with these vibratory properties by paying attention to the details of our lives and to those elements that connect us with natural forces.

Ayurveda and Quantum Theory

At the quantum level life consists of pulses of energy that differ in frequency between life forms and "non-living" matter. At the sub-atomic level we have the same ingredients as a flower, or a bird, a rock or a drop of rain. We have the elements of ether/space, air, fire, water and earth within our bodies in the form of acids, enzymes, fluids, tissues, and the movement and function of muscles and organs. These elements and our pulse of life are sustained by nutrition in the very broadest sense and we get that from food, from our breathing and from the attention we give to ourselves. We flourish when given the right kind of attention and wither when given the wrong kind.

Ayurvedic principles came to us from seers, philosophers and people of wisdom 5000+ years ago, people who were connected to the natural world with an intimacy that might seem hard to achieve nowadays. Using intuition, meditation and the powers of insight, these originators knew the human condition in ways that now seem remarkable. The principles that have come down through the Vedas are, however, more relevant and have more resonance now than ever before. Human beings have reached the point in their development when they have the power to destroy their own origins. We have developed knowledge and technologies that can tamper with genetic structure; we've polluted the atmosphere for 300 years (and to critical levels within the past 80 years) with major climatic change underway; we've slaughtered millions of our own kind in the space of 60 years (and that still continues); and we have all-powerful high speed technology with the capability of mass communication and mass destruction on a global scale. Never-theless, we are still natural beings in a world that though damaged still contains the essence of all that we are and still provides the conditions and resources for life. Our planet is the womb in which we continue to flourish. We forget our natural origins too easily in societies that are overrun with distracting market-driven commodities and influences. It takes concerted effort to even hear the sound of silence in a 100 mph world with television images cutting and changing every 3 seconds, media in every form pouring over us, desperate travelling conditions on over-crowded roads and pressures of every kind piling up around us. This corrosive stew can only lead to breakdown and disaster. Regaining meaningful, constructive contact with our natural resources is critical to the health of the individual and society. It is the most beneficial thing we can do at this moment in the history of the planet.

Ayurveda sees the world in a very similar way to the quantum scientists. Separation is an illusion: the quantum view of energetic connections within the microscopic domains reflects Ayurvedic principles of a holistic universe in which the fundamental elements (particles) of existence are ever present in a vibrational primordial "stew" in which all potential exists. Pulsating energies create existence and create the conditions we experience as we pass through each phase of our consciousness. We are manifestations of a power greater than we understand and have so much more potential than we realise. We are not the captives of a limited worldview or set of external circumstances, our potential is limitless. We are created to be whole and healthy and have the gift of emotional intelligence, intellect and a sense of enquiry to help us feel the full range of human experience and to move our lives forward. These are lofty sentiments, but it is why we are here. Misery, depression and joyless existence are poor options when the alternatives are so much better and within our reach.

A good start is to accept that we are not simply the sum of all our past experiences, or our jobs or our family backgrounds. They have influenced the way we see ourselves and the things around us, but the past only influences us because we allow it to do so. We are all alive now, in this moment, and our power lies in the choices we make now. Choice is a powerful tool but only when linked to knowledge and this begins with knowing our body. All the mental gymnastics in the world, all the intellectual achievements and financial rewards are useless if we don't know who we are and what we need at the most fundamental physical, spiritual and emotional levels. We each have a body and the experience of a physical existence that is our foundation for life. We can make this marvellous gift of a body into something that functions properly and we do that by understanding and working with the factors that immediately influence us. We are a small part of something bigger than us and we can work to be a healthy functioning part of that bigger organism or follow a different path to become a faulty part that functions badly.

We are reflections of the natural world and have, in our cells, the same molecular ingredients as everything around us. We breathe oxygen from an atmosphere that has been sealed and self-contained around our planet for billions of years. The molecules in this special living space have been circulating and re-circulating since life began and we are sharing them with every other living thing and with all life that has gone before us. We eat foods that originate one way or another from soils and seas consisting of the same atoms that have always existed. When we die our bodies will return to that same atomic state and the cycle will continue. We are custodians of a temporary assembly of molecules forming organisms of incredible complexity with the potential to blow the world to pieces or to live in harmony. We might not directly change the world, but we can change ourselves and that will generate incremental change to all around us.

One of the problems affecting most of society is that we have lost our sense of connection to both our immediate surroundings and to nature and the world we live in. We have become insulated against natural influences and conditioned to think we know more than we do. We are human animals with limited vision—other creatures have more powerful vision (some can even see ultraviolet light)— and limited hearing in that we only hear a very limited range of frequencies. Our insular outlook is reinforced because as a species we've been able to develop technologies that enable us to see what we cannot see naturally, thus inflating our sense of omnipotence; but technology does not replace direct experience. What it reveals however, as we have seen in our introduction to quantum physics, is that everything is interconnected. We cannot actually see gravity, but it exists. If we could make gravity visible we would see waves and threads of gravitational energy. Water is everywhere: in the oceans, in our cells and throughout the atmosphere; rivers of vapour flow around the planet. So many things happen that we cannot see, but we are nevertheless a part of what goes on. The notion of empty space between things is an illusion. Everything is connected in ways we simply cannot always detect. The mistake is to believe that we know more than we do and to take interrelatedness with the natural world for granted.

Perceptions have changed, pressurised by mass communication technology and global socio-economic forces. People now lead their lives more separately than ever before. Many societies once knew that everything was connected and honoured this quality. They had a sense of responsibility to the environment that they lived in and to other life forms. They knew that every action had consequences and that life should be respected. In recent centuries that sense of connectedness has been shattered. We now suffer from a loss of place, a loss of the sense that we are a part of something bigger than ourselves, encouraged by technology that removes us from direct experience and also removes us from modes of production that instil thoughtless consumption and separateness. Information bombards us in a deeply fragmented fashion, without context, sense of history or explanation on a twenty-four hour per day basis, at a brain frazzling frequency. Powerful and persistent influences originate from sources that bear no relationship to where and who we are, or even to the community we live in, or to our extended family. We suffer because of this.

For the first time a single species now has the power to alter the biological, physical or geological conditions of life on the planet. As a species, humans are powerfully creative and carelessly destructive. There are more of us than at any time in the planet's history. We have overseen the destruction of our own and other species, together with the natural world on an unprecedented scale that escalates every year. We produce, consume and waste in a way that has never been possible until now, using technologies with the potential for greater impact on the planet's ecosystems than anything before. Consumption seems to define who we are, but everything we consume has to come from somewhere. We aren't creating new materials, simply using up what already exists on the planet, and in the process we are removing materials and life forms that sustain our ecosystem and replacing them with things that damage all that we need for life. We live in artificial habitats under the illusion that we can create whatever we want regardless of the consequences to our planet.

The Five Elements of Ayurveda:
Ether/Space, Air, Fire, Water and Earth

Until recently large percentages of the world population felt their affinity to nature as a tangible aspect of daily life. They knew they were made from the things they ate. Now food is an industrial commodity. The environment is seen as a separate, external element to be managed as we see fit rather than something that is within us. We have forgotten that we are the environment.

We need clean air, clean water and light energy from the sun. Modern life estranges us from these biological roots, but the inescapable fact is that we are animals and we need nature. Each of the elements of nature has qualities that are necessary for life. These qualities are complimentary and work together to sustain the vibrations within our molecular structure. Working with our dosha is the most grass roots and practical activity we can undertake. It is as fundamental as learning to speak. Knowing that we consist of the same ingredients as all life around us and that we simply have a unique blend of those ingredients is a liberating thought. The source of energy that vibrates the strands of the universe is unknown by scientists but is known as God to most religions. We act in faith, knowing that there is a greater power than us and the real mystery of life and of existence remains. What we know is that our building blocks are the five elements of nature, known in Ayurveda as ether/space, air, fire, water and earth. They are in every cell of each of us and, as we mentioned in Chapter 1, the proportions of one to another creates the doshas.

Ether/space

This element is the primordial birthplace of all creation and in Ayurvedic terms our source of connection to the cosmos. All vibrations occur within ether/space, the medium that links every particle of existence, forming our reality and our experience of life. All forces exist in space, the gravitational force, electromagnetic force, the weak force and the strong force, and it allows all possibilities to exist at the most microscopic levels.

At the macroscopic level it is in space that we experience daily life; space occurs around objects and in nature. We say that we "need space" to think and to feel un-pressured and this sense of space affects us more immediately than the other elements. We interact with space as a concept and as a reality. When it is removed from us, when we are confined, we suffer. We need space in our minds to understand things. We see and feel the emptiness of space. It provides the place for air movement to occur and without space we would not hear sounds since sound waves travel through space. Every space within our bodies allows movement of air and fluids, the input of essential elements and the output of sounds, expired gases and waste materials. Space is linked directly to the element of air.

Air

Air permeates our whole body and all the life we encounter on this planet. It wasn't until plants could photosynthesise carbon dioxide and create oxygen that the earth's atmosphere could sustain life. Until then the earth's atmosphere was poisonous, full of carbon dioxide. Plant life converted this gas into the oxygen essential to life as we know it. It is a finite resource that remains in balance as long as plant life is allowed to deliver its gift, creating an atmosphere that is precious and finely encapsulated around our planet. What we do to this atmosphere continues to affect life long after we have gone. Certain elements remain unchanged, for thousands of years. Argon atoms remain unprocessed by our breathing process and go back out into the wider environment to be recycled around the world. In the environmental envelope we inhabit there are molecular elements that have existed since Emperors ruled and Buddha, Jesus Christ and Mohammed. Every breath we take suffuses with every life form into infinity.

Air moves: it has shifting qualities, like the wind, and it can be both strong and weak in its force and effect, from tornado strength to a gentle breeze. Air generates movement in the physical world, causing trees to sway and waves to form, (sometimes to terrifying size). Air movement shifts grains, particles and water, eroding surfaces and it creates roughness and dryness. Air movements carry clouds, shift gasses, micro-organisms and germs. Air has the quality of lightness. Air is life: it is everywhere, in every space. It creates movement through the body and is connected to our sense of touch and of kinetic energy.

Fire

All the energy we use to live, eat and move comes from the chemical energy stored in food. All of that energy came from sunlight. Through photosynthesis, plants convert sunlight into chemical energy in the form of sugars. They store it until we harvest it or animals eat it. All of the energy we produce was originally sunlight stored in fossil fuels. Decayed plant and animal matter fed fossil fuels, and within this marvellous system our planet's rich biodiversity produces the conditions we need to survive.

Fire is central to our existence. It saturates our environment; it is in the earth and the sea and it is in our bodies. Sunlight gives life but in Ayurveda it can also deplete life. Sunlight dries the planet and likewise it dries and enervates our bodies; but we need it to maintain health and SAD (seasonal affective disorder) occurs when we don't have sufficient sunlight. Fire represents chemical transformation within our bodies. We speak of fiery energy and heated minds, alluding to the power of fire to create change. It is also connected with the sense of sight and the ability to achieve clarity.

Water

The element of water is central to our lives. We are composed of at least 60% water by weight, held in place by tissue and fibrous matter. Water sustains every cell in our bodies, which have a self-regulating system for maintaining water levels. Water leaves our bodies through perspiration, urine, breath, and in waste products, and thirst ensures we take more in to replenish our fluid levels. We can live without food for a surprisingly long time, but without water we soon die.

The balance between sunlight, evaporation from the sea, cloud formation, wind movement and rainfall is critical to all life, providing the most important source of nourishment. The oceans are the source of all that we are; the largest single element in every human body comes from those oceans. Massive forces beyond human control originate from this element that covers 70% of the planet, and that coverage is extended by the extent to which water vapour circulates around the envelope of our atmosphere. Water cleanses the ecosystem creating movement and transportation. It rejuvenates, cleanses and detoxifies the body, hydrating every cell, embracing embryonic life within the womb. As a Kapha force it forms the basis for lubrication in our bodies and is the vehicle for chemical transactions, but in excess it can douse our essential Pitta fire. Water moves, earth stills; without water there is no life as we know it. Like air, water connects every living thing on the planet. What we do to water we do to ourselves.

Doctor Masaru Emoto is a graduate of the Yokohama Municipal University and teaches at the Open International University as a Doctor of Alternative Medicine. Through his experiments, which have put him in the forefront of the study of water, Dr. Emoto has proved that thoughts and feelings affect physical reality. By producing different focused intentions through written and spoken words and music and literally presenting it to the same water samples, the water appears to "change its expression." Dr. Emoto discovered that crystals formed in frozen water reveal changes when specific, concentrated thoughts are directed toward them. He found that water from clear springs and water that has been exposed to loving words appears in brilliant, complex, and colourful snowflake patterns. In contrast, polluted water, or water exposed to negative thoughts, forms incomplete, asymmetrical patterns with dull colours; the crystals become damaged and malformed. If emotions can affect water crystals what do they do to our cells?

Earth

Without earth we would not live. Everything comes from the soil in the most profound way, because most of our food comes directly from it. We take food in, break it down and use the molecules to build and re-build what we are. We are created from the molecules that plants and animals have eaten that we then ingest into our own cells. Soil has formed over billions of years of plant and animal decomposition and our earth is a finite resource. The atmosphere enveloping our planet is a thin layer that sustains life; the soil that we live from is even thinner and as critical to life. Earth is our mother; it builds us and deserves reverence. Our physical world, the mountains and rocks, the plains and forests are formed from the earth. Our building resources come from the earth. It is the solid foundation for growth, the fertile soil that feeds life and absorbs death.

In our bodies the element of earth is linked to substance and for being well-grounded. We describe well-grounded, reliable individuals as being the "salt of the earth" and they have a nurturing instinct that holds families and societies together. When mixed with water the earth element creates stable conditions, but in the wrong quantities it becomes heavy and slow. It helps our bodies hold onto things and is connected to the sense of smell.

We are biological creatures. We need clean air, clean water and light energy from the sun. We are also social animals and we need physical contact and connection with each other and with natural life forms around us. This has largely been forgotten by western culture. We belong to the environment that we consume so extravagantly. It is not something outside us, it lives within us and we live within it. We are natural animals and we need the balance of resources that nature has provided for free. Bob Constanza, an ecological economist has calculated that to build systems that would maintain the earth's atmosphere and ecosystems (excluding the millions of pollinating insects) would cost $33 trillion per year. Nature does this for free. Nature provides resources of a financial value many times more than all the economies in the world for free, and yet to governments and economies and to many people who have ignored their natural roots, the environment is external. Economic growth, world travel and wholesale consumption will mean nothing to coming generations who are forced to take defensive measures against the poisoned climate and ruined world we will leave behind unless changes are made. We have to support and renew natural resources such as rain forests, sub-soils and ocean environments. Consumption without renewal devastates our world.

Concerted pressure at grass roots level can begin the process of change necessary to avoid disaster. This begins with how we treat our immediate environment, beginning with our bodies and extending into the places and spaces we inhabit and cherish, and to the touch and care we exchange with loved ones. On a day-to-day basis we meet these needs by interacting with the five elements, by giving attention to ourselves and to each other. We need to place value on things that matter, such as a sense of place, of time and of context. We begin change in the world by changing our own attitudes to whom and what we are.

Chapter 3

The Senses:
Taste, Smell and Sight

Our work on the six senses with Victor, Penelope and Karen provides templates that can be adapted and applied to all dosha combinations. Every one of us is born to experience the world through our senses. Some people have greater facility with certain senses than others, but the ability and willingness to use these gifts lies fully within the reach of everyone. The senses are our direct link with the breadth, variety and intensity of every facet of our environment and without them we lose context, identity and connection with other living things. The pleasure and effort involved in invigorating our senses through self-awareness and Ayurvedic practices is an investment in our quality of life that far exceeds any other conventional form of investment we might make. This work does not guarantee a 10% increase in cash value, more girlfriends or boyfriends, holidays or gadgets. The rewards for the time taken to build and strengthen our senses is far greater than any of these; it goes beyond material benefits and taps into the meaning of our life and our role as sentient beings joining in a continuing process of renewal and creation.

New, frenetic cultural and social customs have replaced the values that were once fundamental to the nuclear family and to societies that had stability and a holistic view of their place in the world. There are now many influences and pressures that blind us to a natural acceptance of the transience of life, to the fact that we are part of a continuum of birth and rebirth. Such pressures ultimately detract from our ability to experience each stage in our journey. These stages are precious opportunities for growth, and involve the accumulation of knowledge and diverse experiences.

We see that each of our three case studies is quite different in physique and temperament. They are each in an unbalanced state, as we have noted from Linda's interviews, and in these states they are experiencing extremes of behaviour, emotions and general health. Their work with their senses and their lifestyles will bring them back into balance. They will still have specific doshas and all the characteristics these entail, but they will have harmony and will feel and look happy and well. They will, in a sense be properly functioning organisms within a larger organism. They have the gift of life with all the range of choice and opportunity that this involves, but they are not independent of the greater creation. They are integral to the life that goes on around them and contribute to it by the attention they give it. They give this greater creation the attention it requires by giving attention to themselves. That is what our senses are for. They enable us to pay attention to every detail of every minute of our existence.

We undergo changes in our passage through life and each one is vital to the health of the greater organism. We are born, we grow, we develop purpose and creative fire, we produce and reproduce, we connect with the universe and we die to begin the cycle of rebirth and re-creation over again. This is the process that we are a part of, one that is shared with every living thing. Ayurveda describes three main stages in life, each one exhibiting the best and balanced characteristics of the three main doshas. Childhood is seen as a Kapha state, when we are grounded, quite literally, in Mother Earth, in the form of our mother and the whole family. During this time we are nurtured and grow, hopefully within a stable environment that allows for the development of our senses and our impression of the world. Adulthood is our Pitta stage. We have acquired knowledge and skills and we have purpose, clarity and the strength and maturity of ego to get things done and to support our families and ourselves. The later years, old age, are our Vata period, when the Vata qualities of ether and air allow us to connect with the universe and prepare for our return to the ultimate state of potential. This is the period when we have the capacity and opportunity for reflection plus the experience and acquired wisdom to contribute to life around us compassionately, without excess ego. We finally enter into a Kapha state, when we once again become grounded as we prepare for a return to the Mother Earth we came from.

This structure has been damaged at societal levels by the spread of industrialized societies and the dissolution of nuclear families. In earlier times, children grew up within extended families supported by adults of varying ages, embraced by energy levels and emotional levels of different intensity, secure in their identity as children on a learning path. Adults worked, developed and created emotional wealth for themselves and their offspring. The elderly contributed to the family with their presence, their mellowness and acceptance of who they were and with their wisdom and sense of spirituality. The elders had no direct responsibility for others and this allowed them the time to develop their inner lives in the light of a lifetime's experiences. Their sense of spirit contributed to the inner life of the family.

That has changed. Now we are persuaded on a daily basis that certain media-led versions of youth are the only ideal to strive for and that age is bad, something to be avoided and denied. Even scientific discourse describes the diminution of senses and abilities with age rather than celebrating the increased perception and spiritual potential that accrue with experience and reflection. True, there are certain cultures in which age is respected more than others, both in Europe, Asia and the Americas, but media pressure is remorseless in its persistence, showing unrealistic and un-attainable images of eternal youthfulness. In those cultures in which age is respected the elders enjoy a longer period of life when they are respected for their attributes.

Unfortunately such recognition of the benefits of aging is rarely found in the western world. Pace, fragmentation and false values have led to imbalanced Vata conditions across the whole of society and a dearth of mature Pitta qualities. Energy created by misplaced societal pressures has inhibited the natural and spiritual capacity of Vata and exaggerated the unbalanced qualities of inflammation, excessive movement and change, waywardness, lack of con-centration and lack of stillness. These are serious losses. In Ayurveda aging is seen as the return to our essential self, when we prepare to die and return to the earth. Our bodies are intended to undergo a slow and gradual process of dissolution; with that comes access to other qualities. In this quieter, less active time we have the opportunity to connect to our inner spirit. This quality of spiritual connection can then be communicated from older members of the family to younger members. If we live our lives connected to our senses we will undoubtedly be better equipped to live our Vata age as we are intended to. It is not natural for us to leap hurdles and high jumps or sprint in this phase, nor is it productive to strive too hard to thwart the aging process. What we gain in old age are the equal blessings of experience and wisdom, of compassion and love. If we haven't taken care of our senses throughout life and used them to their full potential, we will suffer from the imbalanced Vata characteristics of loss of memory, sight and smell, and of the ability to focus on what is important. Fortunately it is never too late to develop our senses and even in old age we can enjoy the benefits achieved from awareness-building work. If we live our adult lives properly connected to our senses, they will be strengthened and we will be better equipped to live the Vata age as fully aware spiritual beings. We will have something great to give to our families and communities; we can teach those in the Pitta stage to listen to our wisdom.

Some work is required to regain our awareness. There is no mystery to this. We simply need to put time and some effort into each of our six senses.

The senses of taste, smell and sight

Taste

Linda began by introducing our three subjects to the six tastes of Ayurveda. They are:

Sweet
Sour
Salty
Pungent
Bitter
Astringent

These tastes are the building block of nutrition. All food falls into one or other of these categories and as we have seen in the two previous chapters, the tastes are closely identified with the five elements in the universe. In Appendix C you will find a comprehensive chart showing a full range of foods and their taste categories, together with a table that indicates which foods are best suited to each dosha. Lists and tables are great aids for speedy access to information and you should use them as much as you need. However it is better that you understand the qualities inherent to the tastes and how they affect an individual's dosha from a practical viewpoint rather than simply relying on the tables. Linda took our three subjects through a process that will also help you to understand your own needs.

Victor, Penelope and Karen were to learn new ways of categorising food that would allow them to reassess what they should be eating and how they should be using food to help balance their physical and emotional lives. Linda showed them that each of the six tastes crosses conventional western food boundaries. They learned that divisions between carbohydrates, proteins, fruits and other products matter less than the food's dryness, moisture, hotness and coldness.

Linda taught Victor that his Vata constitution already consisted of the pungent, bitter and astringent tastes and that if he ate those tastes in any quantity he would simply increase their concentration in his body and knock himself out of balance. What he needed to do was concentrate on the sweet, sour and salty to correct his Vata imbalances. Penelope's Pitta constitution already consisted of sour, salty and pungent tastes and she needed sweet, bitter and astringent tastes to correct her imbalances. Karen's Kapha constitution consisted of sweet, sour and salty tastes and she need to balance herself with pungent, bitter and astringent tastes.

Victor, Penelope and Karen needed to understand why these particular tastes complimented or damaged their doshas. For each of them it was important to realise that their power of digestion was unique to themselves and was not something that fitted easily into a formula. Their digestive fires required appropriate amounts of food of the correct type. Starvation or excess was not the answer and they would learn what their individual requirements were over time. What they needed to do was establish some core principles on which they could base the new nutritional patterns that would encourage their digestive fire to build strength and health. Symptoms such as gas, bloating, irritation, burping, etc., that the three of them experienced at various times indicated nutritional and possibly emotional imbalances that could be tended to and corrected. Eating properly prepared food that complimented each of their doshas would allow their bodily organs to function without hindrance and their constitutions to build and re-build effectively. Most importantly, Linda stressed to each of her three students that insight based upon detailed knowledge of their doshas and the six senses would only come about through practise. They would fully experience the sensory and material elements of life that suited them individually and would over a period of time get to know when they had reached a balanced state and when they were unbalanced. That is half the battle, since most people don't know how they feel with any precision. Victor, Penelope and Karen would bring new knowledge and intuition to bear on their own states of well-being and take the steps necessary to provoke change when required and to sustain improvements once begun.

The Gunas or Qualities

Linda took a step back and got them to look at the gunas, or qualities, that were embedded within their constitutions. In Ayurveda the range of qualities, attributes and characteristics are referred to as gunas. They occur in nature and manifest in specific combinations within our Prakruti or constitution. They are concentrated in different amounts to form our doshas and the same qualities are found in our food. We need the food and the specific tastes that compliment our qualities rather than aggravate them. For instance, a lettuce has particular characteristics that are different from a cabbage or a carrot or an onion even though they are all vegetables and these characteristics are defined within the list of qualities (gunas). Let us look at these qualities before considering tastes and examples of specific foods in greater detail. When we first examined Victor, Penelope and Karen we saw how certain of these qualities were manifested in their doshas. Here is a full list of the qualities and a generalised summary of their attributes. Note that in the context of food, preparation and our mental state also contribute to the qualities. Our mood transfers itself into the food we work with.

Heavy: increases bulk and mass but can cause dullness and lethargy or heaviness. It increases Kapha and decreases Vata and Pitta. Heavy foods include avocado, cheese, banana, urid dhal and many others and they suppress appetite, being difficult to digest. Heavy foods are grounding and strengthening and best eaten in small quantities, since in excess they tax the digestion, creating illness. Strong digestion coupled with vigorous exercise counteracts these tendencies.

Light: helps digestion, reduces bulk and cleanses, creating freshness and alertness but also leading to ungroundendess. It increases Vata and Pitta and decreases Kapha. Light foods are easiest to digest and include lettuce, basmati rice, egg white and many more. They can be taken in larger quantities since they stimulate the digestion.

Slow: creates relaxation and slow action but also increases sluggishness and dullness. It increases Kapha and decreases Vata and Pitta. Slow foods are generally oily and thick.

Sharp: promotes sharpness and a quick understanding of information and situations, with experiences of all kinds having a quick effect on the body, but it also creates ulcers and irritation of the skin, stomach, intestines, eyes, and general disposition and causes excessive fire. It increases Vata and Pitta and decreases Kapha. Sharp foods include chillies and citrus fruits that stimulate digestion in moderation.

Cold: creates numbness and unconsciousness, fear, contraction and insensitivity. It increases Vata and Kapha and decreases Pitta. Cold foods slow and calm the digestion and include milk, coconut, dill, coriander and many more. Cold and hot foods need to be balanced within our diet.

Hot: promotes heat and good digestion, cleansing and expansion, but can also lead to inflammation, anger and hate. It increases Pitta and decreases Vata and Kapha. Hot foods include most spices, chilli, garlic, yoghurt, red lentils, honey and many more. Honey and red lentils have subtle heating qualities that may not be obvious at first.

Oily: creates smoothness, moisture, movement, lubrication and vigour but in excess leads to ingratiating and manipulative behaviour. It increases Pitta and decreases Vata and Kapha. Oily foods help to lubricate the digestive tract and the production of digestive secretions when eaten in moderation, but can inhibit these processes when taken in excess. They include ghee, vegetable oils, animal fats, soya beans and some vegetables.

Dry: increases the absorption of fluids but can lead to increased dryness, constipation and nervousness. It increases Vata and decreases Pitta and Kapha. Dry foods are less beneficial to digestion than oily foods but in moderation can increase digestive fire (agni) and include buckwheat, rye, millet, most beans and dark leafy greens. Such foods require moistening to be easily digested.

Slimy: decreases roughness and increases smoothness and care. It increases Pitta and Kapha and decreases Vata. Slimy foods support lubrication and digestion and include okra and slippery elm bark.

Rough: causes cracking of the skin and bones and creates carelessness and rigidity. It increases Vata and decreases Pitta and Kapha. Rough food tends to move digestion and assimilation through the system, but can be too harsh for some people, particularly Vata types; rough foods include oat, bran, biscuits and dry bread.

Dense: promotes solidity, strength and density. It increases Kapha and decreases Vata and Pitta. Dense foods behave like heavy foods and include unleavened bread and dumplings.

Liquid: promotes salivation and cohesiveness, dissolves and liquefies. It increases Pitta and Kapha and decreases Vata. Liquid foods enhance lubrication and the digestion of carbohydrates in the mouth, and include water and fruit juices.

Soft: creates softness, delicacy, tenderness, relaxation and care. It increases Pitta and Kapha and decreases Vata. Soft foods soothe digestion but can put the digestive fire out when eaten in excess and include tapioca, rice pudding and milk.

Hard: increases strength and hardness but also rigidity, selfishness, callousness and insensitivity. It increases Vata and Kapha and decreases Pitta. Hard foods behave like dense and heavy foods, putting great demands on the digestive fire but building the body, and include nuts and apples

Static: promotes stability, support and faith but can also lead to obstruction and constipation. It increases Kapha and decreases Vata and Pitta. Static foods are similar to gross and cloudy foods in that they inhibit digestive and mental processes, fast food combinations and processed food being typical examples.

Mobile: promotes motion and also movement, restlessness and lack of faith. It increases Vata and Pitta and decreases Kapha. Mobile foods share similar characteristics to subtle and clear foods in that they promote digestive and mental processes and include lettuce, broccoli and light leafy greens.

Subtle: penetrates the capillaries and increases feelings and the experience of emotions. It increases Vata and Pitta and decreases Kapha. Subtle foods, like mobile foods, stimulate the mental and digestive processes and provide accents to other tastes and include lettuce, broccoli and light leafy greens.

Gross: causes obstruction and obesity. It increases Kapha and decreases Vata and Pitta. Similar to static foods, gross foods inhibit digestive and mental processes and include processed and stale or out-of-date food.

Cloudy: reduces penetrating acidity or harshness but can also lead to a lack of perception or clarity. It increases Kapha and decreases Vata and Pitta. Cloudy foods share the same characteristics as static and gross food and include sauces and add-on components to meals.

Clear: pacifies and cleans but also creates isolation and diversion, It increases Vata and Pitta and decreases Kapha. Clear foods share the same characteristics as mobile foods and include water, watermelons and citrus fruit.

We have previously seen in Chapter 1 how the five elements are contained within the six tastes and listed below are the kinds of food that fall within each taste. The tastes cross food boundaries and they have physical and emotional effects on our awareness. A list of tastes and doshas can be found in Appendix C.

Sweet

Sweet tastes are the dominant taste, formed from the **water and earth elements** and especially useful for grounding the fearful nervous energy of Vata. These are cooling tastes, which can be good for the heat of a Pitta type and they inhibit digestion to some extent, especially in excess. The sweet taste occurs in food that is often heavy and moist and it recreates that condition in the body, making it less useful to Kapha types. We should not fall into the trap of thinking of the sweet taste as something that belongs to the domain of ice cream, chocolates, sugars, sweets and pastries. These are artificial concoctions. When found within healthy natural and non-refined food the sweet taste increases bodily tissue and relieves hunger. It is nurturing, nourishing and, in balance, promotes satisfaction, love and a sense of well-being, with the capacity to calm the nervous system. In excess it leads to complacency, inertia and obesity. It does not stimulate digestion but does provide a feeling of satisfaction. This taste occurs in natural sugar, milk, butter, rice, bread, pastas and root vegetables.

Sour

Sour tastes are formed from the **earth and fire elements** and helps digestion and the elimination of wastes. Sour tastes are often found in food that is slightly heavy and moist. They have a mildly warming effect on the body over time and can as a result aggravate certain conditions. They are good for Vata types because of their mild heating qualities, less good for Pitta types who are already heated, and can be too moist and heavy for Kapha types. It is best for Pitta and Kapha to use other tastes to balance sour, whilst Vata digestion benefits from its heaviness, moistness and earthiness. Sour tastes can stimulate and freshen the senses and our awareness, but in excess they can create "sour grapes" or envy. They are the hotter tastes—cheese, tomatoes, vinegar and pickles, citrus fruits, grapefruits and yoghurt.

Salty

Salty tastes are formed from the **fire and water elements** and are useful in small quantities by all types to help cleanse bodily tissues and activate digestion. Food of the salty taste often tends to be slightly moist and heavy (discount the salt we sprinkle too liberally on our food) and is somewhere between sweet and sour in this regard. The fire element gives salt its heating quality that helps digestion when consumed in moderation. It is good for Vata types because of this, less good for Pitta for the same reason and tends to create weight gain through water retention in Kapha types. The salty taste has marked emotional characteristics; it can lead to rigid attitudes and emotional contraction in some and to a desire for instant gratification in others. Sometimes this creates a person who "has to be right all the time." Its use in packaged foods creates that urge to carry on eating more and more of the same stuff. Salty tastes stimulate water retention but do not increase our capacity for weight gain as much as sweet tastes. In moderation salty tastes enhance digestion. In excess they cause waterlogging, irritation and exhaustion, with inflammation of the stomach. They are hot tastes—salt, sauces, salted products, seaweeds, juicy vegetables and tomatoes

Pungent

Pungent tastes are formed from the **elements of air and fire** and are the hottest of the tastes. They help stimulate appetite and digestion and they maintain metabolism and the balance of secretions in the body. Pungent tastes remain hot, light and dry in our bodies throughout the digestive process, making them ideal for Kapha types who benefit from their drying effect. In small quantities they are good for Vata because they stimulate digestion and they are least useful to Pitta types, who need no extra heating up. The pungent taste help to stimulate movement and motivation, and it has a clearing effect on the senses. In excess pungency creates anger and resentment. Pungent balances well with sweet and sour tastes. Pungent is the hottest and driest of the tastes—hot peppers, salsa, ginger, garlic, cloves and hot spices taken in smaller quantities.

Bitter

Bitter tastes come from the **elements of air and space** and can be used by all types in small quantities. It is the coldest and lightest of the tastes and tends to be dry. Bitter detoxifies the blood, controls skin ailments and tones the organs. Bitter continues to have a lightening and drying effect on the body during the whole process of digestion, especially useful for Pitta types and Kapha types in moderation and less useful for Vata types. The bitter taste balances the heavy moist qualities of the sweet, sour and salty tastes and acts as a beneficial accent to most meals. It helps to stimulate clear sightedness and an urge to see through false impressions or situations, but in excess is associated with disillusionment and grief. Bitter is the coldest and driest taste—dark green leafy vegetables, radishes, sprouts, celery, turmeric and spices.

Astringent

Astringent tastes are formed from the **elements of air and earth** and can be used in medicinal quantities by all types. The astringent principle helps to reduce bodily secretions and constricts bodily tissue. It is cooling and has a slight drying quality and is useful to Pitta types because it moderates their heat, to Kapha types because its lightness and dryness balance their heavier qualities and is least useful to Vata types who are already light and dry. Astringency contracts and slows down the digestion and the taste should be used moderately. Medicinal uses of the astringent taste use this constricting quality to promote healing. Astringency encourages a realistic approach to situations and in small quantities it "mops up" extreme emotions. Taken in excess astringency can create a shut down—a loss of interest in anything. Astringent tastes are colder and dry—beans, teas, apples, pomegranates, cranberries, cauliflower, cabbages and dark leafy greens.

The following is a list of the taste categories as they relate to the three main doshas. Remember that each dosha already consists of three tastes and these are the one that don't need reinforcing. If you are hot you don't need more heat, you need gentle cooling; if you are heavy you need lightening; if you are airy and ungrounded you need substance and grounding.

Vata tastes are

Pungent   Pungent tastes are the hottest and driest tastes—hot peppers, salsa, ginger, garlic, cloves and hot spices.

Bitter   Bitter tastes are the coldest and driest—dark green leafy vegetables, radishes, sprouts, celery, turmeric and spices.

Astringent   Astringent tastes are colder and dry—beans, teas, apples, cauliflower, cabbages and dark leafy greens.

Vata types should eat less of the above as they aggravate Vata problems

Vata types should favour

Sweet   Sweet tastes are nurturing and cooling—natural sugar, milk, butter, rice, bread, pastas and root vegetables.

Sour	Sour tastes are the hotter tastes—cheese, tomatoes, pickles, citrus fruits, grapefruits and yoghurt.
Salty	Salty tastes are hot tastes—salt, sauces, salted products, sea weeds, juicy vegetables and tomatoes.

Vata types should favour more warm, oily, heavy foods.

Pitta tastes are

Sour	Sour tastes are the hotter tastes—cheese, tomatoes, pickles, citrus fruits, grapefruits and yoghurt.
Salty	Salty tastes are hot tastes—salt, sauces, salted products, sea weeds, juicy vegetables and tomatoes.
Pungent	Pungent tastes are the hottest and driest tastes—hot peppers, salsa, ginger, garlic, cloves and hot spices.

Pitta types should eat less of the above as they aggravate Pitta problems

Pitta types should favour

Sweet	Sweet tastes are nurturing and cooling—natural sugar, milk, butter, rice, bread, pastas and root vegetables.
Astringent	Astringent tastes are colder and dry—beans, teas, apples, cauliflower, cabbages and dark leafy greens.
Bitter	Bitter tastes are the coldest and driest—dark green leafy vegetables, radishes, sprouts, celery, turmeric and spices.

Pitta types should favour cooler foods of medium weight and cooler liquids.

Kapha tastes are

Sweet	Sweet tastes are nurturing and cooling—natural sugar, milk, butter, rice, bread, pastas and root vegetables.
Sour	Sour tastes are the hotter tastes—cheese, tomatoes, pickles, citrus fruits, grapefruits and yoghurt.
Salty	Salty tastes are hot tastes—salt, sauces, salted products, sea weeds, juicy vegetables and tomatoes.

Kapha types should eat less of the above as they aggravate Kapha problems

Kapha types should favour

Pungent	Pungent tastes are the hottest and driest tastes—hot peppers, salsa, ginger, garlic, cloves and hot spices.
Bitter	Bitter tastes are the coldest and driest—dark green leafy vegetables, radishes, sprouts, celery, turmeric and spices.
Astringent	Astringent tastes are colder and dry—beans, teas, apples, cauliflower, cabbages and dark leafy greens.

Kapha types should favour more light, dry and warm food.

Taste for a Vata person. Linda had already gone into detail on the kinds of food Victor needed but they looked again and summarised things. He needed food from Linda's list of sweet, sour and salty tastes. These would keep him balanced and although he could have samples or accents of the other tastes he needed to base his diet around those three. What really made an impact on Victor was Linda's description of the healing power of taste. Without the range of tastes in his diet Victor had been undergoing sensory deprivation. Worse than that, so much food that's available from the supermarkets is smothered with synthetic flavours and excessive salt and sugar that mask the sheer lack of real building qualities from true, natural tastes. Victor could see that there was a real choice to be made that would change his health in a big way.

... and for a Pitta person. Penelope had by now got the idea that as a Pitta she needed sweet, astringent and bitter tastes. Because she already had sour, salty and pungent tastes within her Pitta constitution, she couldn't afford to increase their properties, which is exactly what she had been doing with the food she'd been eating. The correct tastes from Linda's list would have an immediate impact on her anger, heat and stress levels. There were lots of options to go for and Linda's weekly Ayurvedic cookery sessions got her onto the right track. Like Victor, without the balance of correct tastes in her diet she had not only been undergoing sensory deprivation, but she had, effectively, been throwing petrol on a fire with all those hot tastes and her Pitta constitution. Not only that, the ice-cold citrus drinks she consumed were too acidic and too cold for a heated person to take. She needed fluids at room temperature otherwise her Pitta fire would steam up from sudden intakes of cold fluid. The

Tapas and the curries might have been alright had she avoided the really spicy variations, but Penelope had got into the habit of ordering hot food, just as she habitually ate cheese and pickled foods at lunch.

... and for a Kapha person. Karen understood the position she had got herself into and whilst healthy for some, her diet of dairy products, bread, grains and sweet and sour tastes, combined with a high fluid intake, was guaranteed to slow her down and create weight gain. The sweet tastes are good for building mass and strength, great for Vata and Pitta but Karen was a naturally well-built woman. Sour tastes in Karen's case came from dairy products and salty tastes create fluid retention, so she had been systematically slowing herself down from the inside out! She never actually overate and was certainly not a binge eater and yet her size was something she was uncomfortable with and she dieted to combat a gradual increase in weigh over several years. Once again Linda was able to lead Karen to the best situation for her body type. Karen required pungent, bitter and astringent tastes because she was already sweet, sour and salty. Everything she'd been eating fell into the wrong category and she had paid the penalty with weight gain, lethargy and low energy levels. She spent years increasing the natural tastes of her own body type and not taking in the benefits that a spicier diet would provide. Luckily for Karen her Kapha body type suited all spices so her options were quite unlimited, although she needed to watch her salt intake.

They looked at the sense of smell

Smell is considered to be one of two chemical senses (the other being taste), so-called because chemicals are involved in the transfer of information between molecules and our sensory receptors. With this sense we sample our environment for information. We are continuously testing the quality of the air we breathe (this will alert us to potential dangers, e.g. smoke) as well as using this sense to inform us of other relevant information, such as the presence of food or another individual. The chemicals detected by our sensory systems need to have certain properties. For instance, odour molecules must be small enough to be volatile (less than 300–400 relative molecular mass) so that they can vapourise, reach the nose and then dissolve in the mucus. This tells us that smell, unlike taste, can signal over long distances (an early warning device). We appear to have an innate ability to detect bad, aversive smells and even one-day old babies give facial expressions that indicate rejection when given fish or rotten egg odour.

Our sense of smell serves a recognition function. We all have our own unique smell, some more pleasant than others, and can recognise and be recognised by it. Children can distinguish between the smell of their siblings and other children of the same age and babies and mothers recognise each other's smell. Emotion can be communicated by smell and we know that dogs and horses are very sensitive to the smell of fear in humans. Recent research has shown that a panel of women can discriminate between armpit swabs taken from people watching "happy" and "sad" films (men were less good at this). The emotions of others, for example fear, contentment, sexuality, may therefore be experienced and communicated by smell. Smell, memory and the other senses are intimately connected.

The social behavior of most animals is controlled by smells and other chemical signals. Dogs and mice rely on odours to locate food, recognize trails and territory, identify kin and find a receptive mate. Social insects, such as ants, send and receive intricate chemical signals that tell them precisely where to go and how to behave at all times of day. Humans are less connected to their sense of smell and they "see" the world largely through eyes and ears. We neglect the sense of smell—and often suppress our awareness of what our nose tells us. Many of us have been taught that there is something shameful about odours and yet the smells that surround us affect our well-being throughout our lives.

Smell and memory

Countless studies have shown that recall can be enhanced if learning was done in the presence of an odour and that same odour is presented at the time of recall. Work by Walter Freeman (Freeman, 1991) has shown that smell memory is context-dependent and can be modified in the light of new experience, implying that our olfactory sense is continuously dynamic, updating as we live and experience new things. We can, in fact, work with our sense of smell to shift moods and feelings deliberately. Odour memory falls off less rapidly than other sensory memory and it lasts a long time, providing a strong foundation within which we can embed our increased perceptive ability.

We have all experienced the powerful effects of smell and memory in combination. Smells retain an uncanny power to move us. A certain food smell, cigar smoke or a long-forgotten scent can instantly conjure up scenes and emotions from the past.

In *The Remembrance of Things Past,* French novelist Marcel Proust powerfully described what happened to him after drinking a spoonful of tea in which he had soaked a piece of madeleine (a type of cake). Proust noted that seeing alone was not enough. He needed to taste and smell the madeleine. In this evocative and influential novel Proust's reference to both taste and smell are so potent because most of the flavour of food comes from its aroma, which wafts up the nostrils to cells in the nose and also reaches these cells through a passageway in the back of the mouth.

Although all of the senses help us to create the full experience of life, smell is often the most underrated and underused sense. Some estimates suggest we can distinguish around 10,000 different smells. How we smell, why we smell and the impact of smell on our everyday life is poorly understood by the scientific community as yet, but in Ayurveda we believe that our sense of smell can be trained and enhanced through attention and focused effort. Unconscious smell memories create powerful links to emotions and to critical elements of our underlying sense of who we are, since taste and smell are so powerfully linked. Without smell, taste is lessened considerably. This is why Linda worked so persistently on this sense with our three case studies. We can work with this sense in order to create intentional changes of moods. Even at a mundane level it is a recognised fact that a sale is more likely if the smell of freshly baked bread permeates a house, such is the power of that "homely" signal. Childhood memories are triggered instantly by certain smells, with all the emotions they contain. We under-estimate the importance of smell to our well-being and although mainstream science is just beginning to recognise that smell can influence mood, memory, emotions, mate choice, the immune system and the endocrine system (hormones), within Ayurveda the influence of smell is intrinsic to the development of the individual. We know that we can communicate by smell—often without knowing it—and that the sense of smell is at the mind-body interface.

Therapy using smell memory

Smells can be put to therapeutic advantage and the medical establishment is investigating this. If smell were to be associated with a positive, healing treatment then the smell itself can substitute for the treatment once the link has been reinforced. If we smell (or taste something) before a negative experience, that smell (or taste) is linked to that experience. The memory is very robust and this can be a problem for unpleasant medical treatments, or surgery when the last meal is often associated with the pain or trauma. The converse also applies and is especially relevant to our work in Ayurveda. It is vital that we build into our olfactory memory banks the association between natural food, properly prepared with spices and herbs, for their healing and building qualities; it is vital that we smell natural odours to embed our affinity with the natural world into our cellular structure; it is vital that we renew and refresh these smell memories by bringing these odours into our homes and working environments using essential oils and other natural fragrances.

We use our senses of sight, touch and hearing unconsciously because we cannot see without open eyes, we cannot easily shut off our hearing and every physical movement stimulates touch. These senses are engaged for most of the time. As a society we have become accustomed to a limited range of smells and tastes and the act of giving attention to these particular senses elicits a disproportionately greater response in our bodies. We need to make conscious efforts to increase our capacity to smell and taste but those efforts are worthwhile. The quality of life improves immeasurably.

Linda spent time with all three of our case studies covering the sense of smell in a general fashion, since there were principles that all three could adapt to their individual regimes. Simple, conscious acts and processes can bring about major change and these specific acts build awareness and create the right circumstances for healing and renewal. Uniquely, smell connects us with our memories and our immediate environment. Smells can take us on an emotional journey more quickly than any other sense. A smell takes us back to the source of when we first experienced it, without effort. The clinical smell of a hospital or the dentist always remains with us and if our experiences were painful, so is the emotional connection we make with that smell. Certain odours, such as the smell of new mown grass or freshly dug soil, or that of freshly baked bread, resonate throughout our lives and cut deeply across cultural boundaries. They establish a state of mind and an expectation of certain conditions, such as a summer's day or a special or festive occasion. These and other odours are familiar enough to recall and are instantly recognised. We usually have more trouble in identifying odours in everyday life and it is in these grey areas that we can locate and extend our sense of smell to develop greater awareness of more elements in our environment. Regardless of our dosha we have to practise in order to heighten our sense of smell. Until we increase our receptivity to a wider range of smells the beneficial effects of this sense will not be fully felt.

In Ayurveda the prime source of healing initiated by smell can be found through the act of food preparation. Thinking about, choosing and preparing food stimulates all of the senses, but smell requires additional attention. Linda took Victor, Penelope and Karen through a demonstration of cutting and slicing a range of foods, including root vegetables such as potatoes, swedes, parsnips, sweet potatoes, carrots and then other vegetables including onions, broccoli, cauliflower, courgettes and capsicums. As she sliced each one Linda got them to smell the differences between each vegetable before and after it was sliced. She got them to breathe deeply and absorb the special character that each vegetable revealed as it was opened up and all three realised the limits they had unwittingly imposed upon themselves in the past through the lack of time and attention they had given to these simple acts. Each one thought they knew what these familiar vegetables would smell like, but opening them up and taking time with them revealed layers of smell that none of the group expected. Linda introduced spices and herbs. Coriander and turmeric had sharply contrasting qualities; one had sweetness and lightness the other deep earthy quality with a bitter edge. Cloves and ginger had keen, pungent smells whilst cabbage had an earthiness that was also astringent.

As Linda took them through a range of food types, all three of them began to realise the constraints they had unknowingly placed on their appreciation of natural food. They also realised how limited their vocabulary of smells was, as is the case with most people until they consciously develop this sense. We don't have the words to describe the drama and mystery of smell until we learn them and experience the differences. When Linda made them smell processed foods their aromatic coarseness and lack of subtlety was apparent. The kitchen was soon seen to be an ideal training ground for noses, the key factor being the quality of attention that one gives to each act of preparation and the time one gives to each item of food. Cooking opened up new aromas and, regardless of dosha, the importance of spices and herbs as agents of transformation and change became obvious. Herbs and spices have particular healing qualities that are initiated by aroma and continue throughout digestion, so it was important to experience their aroma. Cooking smells open up emotional channels, preparing the body for pleasure and, depending upon the food types and one's dosha, for the experiences of calmness, stimulation and perception.

Building upon the notion of practise and experience Linda took Victor, Penelope and Karen outside, on a walk through the local area. Developing perception is often an exercise in slowing down and taking the time to experience the familiar in a different way. We take most things for granted most of the time. A commonly used expression that sums this up is "we walk around with our eyes shut." This implies that we become blind to our surroundings, blasé even, and it can be a truism for the way most people live most of their lives. Awareness and enhanced perception take time and effort and for a large percentage of our lives we think we don't have the energy to give attention to everything that goes on. We filter things out in order to survive and to some extent this is a necessary process. Driving, jogging or walking down the street are activities of differing levels of complexity that require us to concentrate on certain tasks in sequence to achieve success. When doing this we don't do other things. When we drive we don't read anything other than road signs and our car's instruments. There are thousands of things going on in the world outside the car but we learn to pay attention only to certain stimuli. Jogging requires us to look out for things we are liable to run into, such as lampposts, kerbs and pedestrians. Walking requires the least attention to obstacles and more opportunities for reflection and watching the scenery. With some activities we trade off certain kinds of awareness in favour of an enhanced capacity to observe critical elements imposed by that activity.

What Linda wanted them to do on their walk was let go of the perceptual filters they had each become used to and re-learn the art of observation. Once again, as in her demonstration in the kitchen, Linda taught them that the key lay with attention. It's been said before that the average human being can recognize up to 10,000 separate odors. Also, odorant molecules emanating from trees, flowers, earth, animals, food, industrial activity, bacterial de-composition and other humans surround us. Yet when we want to describe these odors, we often resort to crude analogies: something smells like a rose, smells like sweat, or smells like ammonia. Our culture places such low value on olfaction that we have never developed a proper vocabulary for it. In *A Natural History of the Senses*, poet Diane Ackerman notes that it is almost impossible to explain how something smells to someone who hasn't smelled it. There are names for all the pastel tints in a hue, she writes—but none for the tones and tints of a smell. Prompted by Linda, Victor, Penelope and Karen began to realise that whilst they might not yet re-write their vocabulary of smells they could begin to experience them more fully, and if that meant using comparisons such as "smells a bit like..." this or that odour, then so be it. The important thing was to use their sense of smell.

As they began their walk they passed some large rubbish bins left out for collection. Nobody wanted to linger, but Linda drew the three of them to the smells of rotting food that you always find coming from any pile of domestic rubbish. Organic materials decay and they produce a characteristic smell. We recoil from it, partly as a safety response, its unpleasantness keeping us away from the inevitable germs associated with decaying matter. Rotting flesh, vomit and excrement produce smells that warn us of their inherent danger and we don't need to learn that response, it comes naturally. Because we spend most of our lives keeping away from such aromas we remain sensitised to them. If we were to concentrate on them our sensitive reactions would be lessened, although we would always recognise such odours as intrinsically dangerous or unhealthy. The nearest we come to such de-sensitising in daily life is when we change our children's nappies, and we do that out of love!

They set out for a local park. On the way they passed under a canal bridge. The dank, stone walls of the bridge were green with moss and in places dripped with water from the road above. The wet streaks were slimy and rusty looking. Linda got them to stop and breathe in the air in this confined space. The canal was still, the water dark and dirty, not a place to swim. The air was musty and smelled vaguely of decomposing vegetables. Close up the moss and slime were more pungent and smelled completely different from the drier stones of the bridge, which was curved and vaulted, covering them in a long arch that kept out the fresh air from outside. Victor remembered times as a boy when he used to climb along the stone capping of canal embankments and the time when he fell in the water. His friends dragged him out, tearful and stinking, afraid to tell his mum what had happened and unable to get rid of the smell that even now brought up in him a sense of dread and guilt. He'd always been told not to go near those places but he did what boys do and ignored his parents and broke the rules. It was a vivid memory that came in an instant and stirred his emotions.

The park was a short walk away and was enclosed by trees. There were hawthorns in blossom (smelling sweetly with a fragrance that belied their gnarly twisted profiles), birches, some taller beech trees and a scattering of oaks. A long brick wall enclosed one side of the park and against the wall and hemmed in by oak and beech were clusters of rhododendron and dwarf birches, saplings and undergrowth. The open spaces were grassy and hilly and a brook ran through a small valley that wound through the park and vanished towards nearby buildings. Linda took them into the undergrowth and they dug up fresh soil and breathed in its powerful and evocative aroma. It resonated within each of them with an almost primitive pulse. Penelope had never focussed on this kind of aroma before. As a child and teenager she had always been keen on sports but this hadn't involved the kind of earthy adventures that some young people take part in. Her adventures had taken place in relatively organised surroundings and she had missed the childhood opportunities to invent games and play in the muddy dark places. These earthy aromas were very powerful for her. To Victor these smells were like coming home; they took him back to childhood games and adventures that were about as distant from his current experiences as they could be. Unlike Penelope he knew these aromas, but like her he now spent all his time far removed from such sources. These fresh earthy aromas were totally different from the smell of dirt and decay from the rubbish bins. The moist soil and heavy clay smelled of potential and growth.

Over in the park a man mowed the rolling grassy slopes and the wafting contrasts between the light sweet fragrance of the grass and the heavy smelling soil was rich and evocative. They were stopped in their tracks. Penelope and Victor were intoxicated but Karen was less so. She was uncomfortable with the dirt and dampness. She loved Victor's descriptions of his childhood games, but she had hardly ever played with gangs of other kids and had never been especially active at school, when this kind of experience would have happened. She thought the smells of grass and blossom were pleasant but wasn't as enthusiastic about them as the other two.

They smelled the leaves of each bush, noticing subtle differences and realising how difficult it is to describe smells without analogy. Linda explained that this didn't matter; names were less important than experiences and the broad descriptions of "earthy, tangy, fresh, floral, light, heavy, sharp, penetrating, intense, pungent and acidic" mattered more to them at this stage. Linda wanted them to begin to feel the smells and to know what helped them and what hindered them. There were lemony smells and peppery smells and waxy leaves that reminded them of avocado. Some of the smells provoked a taste response and others didn't, but Linda wanted them to do some homework on the association of smells and tastes to get the best out of their taste buds later on.

A small rocky outcrop and some boulders formed a feature in the middle of the park and they went over to it. The rock was cool and rough. Lichen grew on parts of the surface, forming a bright contrast to the surrounding grey and sandy colours. The rock and lichen had separate aromas and the three of them sensed a sweetness from the lichen and different smells between the clefts in the rock and the exposed surfaces. All the aromas were softer and subtler than they expected.

They left the park along a narrow alleyway lined with bushes that were dusty from the passing traffic on the main road close by. The road was slightly above the level of the alleyway and heavy fumes pressed down on them, bitter and toxic. They all had a natural urge to protect their lungs by closing their mouths tightly, screwing up their faces and breathing through noses that immediately reacted to these corrosive gases. Their senses prickled.

The sense of smell for a Vata person. It had all started to make sense to Victor by now and the need to ground his Vata airiness meant that he needed earthy, sweet, floral smells. The smell of the sea was great for him, as were sandalwood and frankincense essential oils, basil and heavy earthy smells, as well as heady sweet floral smells such as jasmine and some roses. Whilst Victor may not become a gardener, the smells of gardening would be very stabilising for him and Linda showed him how to bring them into his life. Sandalwood oil would be good for massage; this and other essential oils, heated over a small burner that he would buy would be a great step forward in making his flat a place that would really cosset him. It was also vital that he concentrated on the sense of smell when cooking.

The sense of smell for a Pitta person. Penelope was similar to Victor in that sweet and earthy smells would be good for grounding her Pitta fire, with floral smells like rose and jasmine, as well as vanilla and lavender, being especially beneficial. Reflective country walks out of the heat of the day and cool evening walks under moonlight would provide opportunities to locate her sense of smell in contexts that would nourish her and stimulate greater awareness and she too needed to take these smells into her home by using essential oils in a burner.

The sense of smell for a Kapha person. Karen's need for livelier and more edgy experiences than she'd been used to showed itself here in the need for citrus and spicy herbal smells. She needed to move away from some of the floral smells she'd used as perfumes and around the house and use tangy fragrances that would lift and stimulate her spirits and shift her awareness. Unlike the other two she didn't need cosseting and she was already grounded because of her Kapha disposition. Risks and edginess were the order of the day from Linda.

They looked at the sense of sight

Our background and the experiences we have affect our attitudes and the way we interpret the things we see around us. Visual education from our school and college days, cultural factors throughout our lives and the all-pervasive daily impact of the media has powerful and persuasive effects on the way we all see the world. We develop learned responses to a range of cultural codes that influence our ideas of beauty, grandeur, harmony, proportion, imbalance, excess, contrast and all of the elements of our natural and built environments. There are however, underlying structural factors that go deeper than the immediate cultural and societal influences. A sense of order and harmony is not simply an advertising executive's bright idea; it already exists within each of us at a cellular level. As products of the natural world we are hardwired with factors for cellular growth and development that exist across nature. Our physical surroundings reflect the proportions, colours, contrasts of light and shade, balances of hard and soft, rough and smooth—and the ratios of scale that exist within us—and we cannot help but respond. For instance, consensus of opinion on the physical beauty of the human form spreads across cultures and centuries, as do concepts of natural beauty in landscape, the fine and decorative arts, architecture and what we now think of as product design. What previous generations and what our contemporaries see as "beautiful" stand the test of time, with some exceptions which prove the rule.

Setting cultural codes, fashions and tastes aside we can acknowledge the beauty, balance and effectiveness of artefacts and images from other times and places because we carry within us a pre-determined sense of harmony and proportion. This pervades our response to every space we encounter, to everything we see and touch and every visual stimulus in our lives. When we are aware, when our eyes are open, we can choose to open up to visual beauty and move away from disharmony and ugliness. Even when our eyes are metaphorically closed these visual influences affect us because our whole body feels the beneficial effects of harmonious forces. We "see" according to our moods and state of mind, but even in a quantum world of shifting states and elements we unconsciously use a series of reference points that remain constant to ground us.

This sense of order can be seen in the classical influences that pervade our culture, be it Western or Eastern. The content of our visual influences may vary, with clear differences between narrative realism in painting, geometric decorative themes, religious symbolism, native cultural artefacts, modernist architecture, photography, fashion, etc., but these examples, which at first glance appear to bear no relation to one another, are connected by the mechanisms behind the seeing eye. The connection between these apparently disparate components is the Golden Mean, a mathematical proportion that describes the ideal ratio within nature. The Golden Mean is a ratio which results in the number "phi" which is 1.61803. To achieve this we take a line and divide it so that the ratio of the large piece (B) to the whole line is the same as the ratio of the small piece (C) to the larger piece (B). A = 161.8% of B and B = 161.8% of C. See Appendix D for an illustration of these ratios.

This ratio occurs throughout nature, in growth patterns in plants, in the ratio of joints in the human body, the proportions of the face, length of limbs to body to overall height, in musical scales, patterns of population growth, mathematics and geometry—in every aspect of life and even in the geometry of planets and the universe. Its use started as early as the design of the great pyramids in Egypt; the Greeks knew it as the Golden Section and used it for beauty and balance in the design of architecture; Renaissance artists knew it as the Divine Proportion and used it in fine and applied art; it can be seen in many great works of architecture, from Notre Dame to the works of Le Corbusier and most 20th and 21st Century architects; it can be seen on every newspaper and magazine page, every gallery space, window displays and the whole of the graphic arts, in the design and layout of public spaces, within great landscape views and in portrait photography the world over, in fact wherever humans exercise choice and visual discrimination we usually find the magic ratio of "phi" or the Golden Mean in evidence. How it is applied can be difficult to conceptualise as the ratio 1.61803. This is too abstract for most of us to relate to and the easiest way to understand its meaning is to think in terms of division of space and form into ratios of 5, 3 and 2. The things we respond to most positively can be divided into these proportions.

Fibonacci Series

Leonardo Fibonacci was an Italian mathematician who, in the 12th Century, introduced decimalisation to Europe in the form of the numbers 0 to 9 and developed what became known as the Fibonacci sequence. This is number sequence is generated by adding the previous two numbers in the list together to form the next and so on and so on... 1, 1, 2, 3, 5, 8, 13, 21, 34, 55 ...

Divide any number in the Fibonacci sequence by the one before it, for example 55/34, or 21/13, and the answer is always close to 1.61803. This is also the Golden Ratio, and hence Fibonacci's Sequence is also called the Golden Sequence. It can be found in the growth patterns of cells and larger forms throughout nature and is the common factor linking rabbit populations, cauliflowers and snails, seed growth, human population growth, the proportions of the human body—the list is endless. See Appendix D for a diagram demonstrating the Fibonacci sequence.

Examples of Fibonacci numbers can be seen in the arrangement of seeds on flower heads and the spiraling growth patterns of leaves around a plant stem. In seed heads the Fibonacci sequence creates arrangements that form an optimal packing of seeds so that, no matter how large the seed head, by following the mathematical progression of the sequence they are uniformly packed at any stage. All the seeds, being the same size, suffer no crowding in the centre and are not too sparse at the edges. Although seeds are usually round or spherical we see them forming hexagonal arrangements on seed heads. This is because hexagonal symmetry is the best general packing arrangement for most circular units and for circular seeds too.

Many plants show the Fibonacci numbers in the spiraling arrangements of the leaves around their stems. If we look down on a plant, the leaves are often arranged so that leaves above do not hide leaves below. This means that each gets a good share of the sunlight and catches the most rain to channel down to the roots as it runs down the leaf to the stem. The Fibonacci numbers occur when counting both the number of times we go around the stem, going from leaf to leaf, as well as counting the leaves we meet until we encounter a leaf directly above the starting one. A typical example of the Fibonacci numbers can be found in the spiralling arrangement of a pine cone's segments.

Nature seems to use the same pattern to place seeds on a seed head that it uses to arrange petals around the edge of a flower *and* to place leaves round a stem. What is more, *all* of these maintain their efficiency as the plant continues to grow. This is a remarkable achievement within a single process. The amazing thing is that a single fixed angle can produce the optimal design no matter how big the plant grows. So, once an angle is fixed for a leaf, that leaf will least obscure the leaves below and be least obscured by any future leaves above it. Similarly, once a seed is positioned on a seed head, the seed continues out in a straight line pushed out by other new seeds, but retaining the original angle on the seed head. No matter how large the seed head, the seeds will always be packed uniformly on the seed head.

And all this can be done with a single fixed angle of rotation between new cells. The principle of a single angle-producing uniform packing, no matter how much subsequent growth occurs, was only proved mathematically as recently as 1993 by Douady and Couder, two French mathematicians. The fixed angle of turn is "Phi" cells per turn or phi turns per new cell.

Analysis of faces and bodies across cultural boundaries using measurements based on Fibonacci and the Golden Section show that those most commonly thought to be beautiful consistently showed evidence of this ratio. Given the evidence of this incredible natural structuring mechanism that seems to underpin most life forms, how can we: a) accept its influence and work with it through choice, when appropriate; b) recognise the best ways to use it; and c) understand how to work with it when we or our surroundings go out of balance. Any principle of organisation is only useful as a guide and our tastes and preferences are also important in building a sense of well-being that arises from our whole lifestyle and environment. Nevertheless, structures provide reference points against which we can check our actions and decision. Our three client's experiences offer great insights into how to use the Golden Mean to our benefit.

The sense of sight for a Vata person. Victor's work in the media industry involved days spent in stimulating and visually active surroundings, travelling to and from work daily through busy traffic. The travelling made him anxious; he always fretted about being late and he always felt strained by the effort of concentrating on everything that went on. In the studio he made critical design decisions on an hourly basis—that was his job, but in doing so over several years he had started to saturate himself with too much information. Information bombards everyone to the extent that a conscious effort is required to select what external influences we want to shut out. We need filters. Victor was typically Vata in the way he responded to everything with enthusiasm and energy, almost without discrimination, and he had a highly developed visual sense that was a genuine asset. In one sense seeing beauty or potential everywhere was a very positive attribute and one of the factors that fed his creative outlook, but the problem was one of context. He was poor at filtering the stimuli that came his way and had a real struggle to organise his thoughts, actions and resources. This aspect of his personality, and the highly charged visually active environments he inhabited, were over-stimulating him. His flat was decorated in strong colours and the surroundings of his social life, from the gym to clubs and bars were all quite intense and he lived his life almost entirely within the built environment.

It was obvious that most of the time he experienced very few natural influences yet they are precisely what a Vata person needs to keep them on Planet Earth. As a Vata type, Victor was full of space and air. Physically and emotionally he was in constant motion and he needed to ground himself with earthy imagery. There were enough hard, rough and changing visual elements around him, ranging from the internet, the office, the traffic and his current domestic surroundings to his social activities, and he needed to slow down the flow of his visual sense and find some structure and stability to rest and renew his sensory banks.

It's one of those 21st Century mantras that we all need to keep in touch with nature, but Victor really did need to see natural colours, textures and images more than most. Being within landscapes and seascapes would be great therapy for him and while he might not always be able to get out into nature, using natural colours in his workplace and at home was essential to the re-building process. He needed to receive the benefits of natural order without the speed of change he suffered from. Feeling and seeing transitions of natural light and colour would re-tune his system. Architectural stability and interior spaces that can be found in cathedrals, churches and galleries and, surprisingly, some of the minimalist modern spaces were also good places for calming his senses. Vata types can balance their high velocity mental activity by placing themselves in ordered and structured environments. The horizontal and vertical planes of landscape and architecture create an immediate feeling of stability in the viewer. Victor didn't need wild scenes with trees blasted by wind and waves smashing onto rocky outcrops. Beautiful though that kind of scene is, it could wait until later as far as he was concerned. In his current state of mind he needed stillness. Linda looked at new colour schemes for his flat, with desert, sky and sea colours being the best options. She showed him how he could use photographs and themes from natural sources to inspire his choices, and how small details such as flowers, grasses and woven fabrics would integrate his senses of sight and touch. These small touches could be taken into his working environment as grounding featured amidst the chaos.

The sense of sight for a Pitta person. Penelope's working life had some positive visual stimulation but revolved mainly around corridors, classrooms and offices that were functional rather than creative. Overflowing desks, notice boards and filing cabinets alternated with pigeonholes and teeming corridors to form the backdrops to her life at school. Because of the inherent rate of change there was very little by way of harmonious visual feedback. Her colleagues in the art department were better off because their students' work was always on display; but teachers move through shifting landscapes and, like Victor, Penelope experienced no stabilising visual imagery on a regular basis. This had created a vicious circle for her: she had become comfortable living in a hothouse atmosphere and regarded pace and intensity as the normal conditions of life. Her home environment was filled with vivid colours, textures and mementos from her travels which were good in a creative sense, but too over heated for her Pitta type; and her recreational activities took her into mechanically styled surroundings, such as the gym, or spotlight club settings which were aggressively styled, with no soothing characteristics whatsoever. Penelope was surprised at the extent to which these extremes had crept into her existence. Her world alternated between utilitarian humdrum working surroundings, with peaks of stressful and often manic activity, and then intense but inappropriate visual and tactile stimulation outside work. She needed visual influences that would calm and cool her Pitta fire.

Like Victor she had no natural imagery to sustain her around home and work and none of the calming, cooling influences that Pittas required. Like him, her natural roots required strengthening but from a slightly different starting point. Penelope needed to see and feel the tranquillity provided by beaches, forests and lakes, the balance and proportion of sky and horizon that would calm her intense Pitta mind. She needed the feeling of structure we get from looking through a camera viewfinder at a beautiful scene and surroundings that would encourage a meditative frame of mind. Pitta types benefit from dark evenings under a cool moon, or from being in the presence of moving water with its soothing natural rhythm, combined with the slower pace of walking though landscape. Whereas Vata types, because of their changeable nature, require time without movement, Pitta types like Penelope benefit from evenly paced, steady walking rhythms, and the sense of space, distance and natural geometry to be found within landscape and seascapes. She needed light and sunshine, but not intense heat, and colour from the cooler end of the spectrum. She needed the textures, colours and tones of forests and grass, the pale tones of sand, and naturally eroded rocky surfaces.

Linda suggested that she might interest her boyfriend in taking her with him on some of his mountain trips instead of focussing her physical activity in gyms. Subtle cooling colours should be brought into her home surroundings and at work too wherever possible, so changes to colour scheme were called for. At home it would be easy to change to cooling blues, greens and also black and white which are good for Pitta and Penelope could bring in imagery of mountains, seas and lakes that would help create small refuges of tranquillity. The natural colour combinations could also be taken into her wardrobe.

The sense of sight for a Kapha person. There were real differences between Karen's experiences and those of Victor and Penelope. Karen's dull working surroundings contrasted with the colourful decorative chaos of her home and what she learned from Linda was how much she needed to stimulate herself with the right balance of visual influences combining colour, tone and contrast.

Kaphas already have stable foundations and Karen could afford to be bold and take some risks. A Kapha type is naturally grounded and solid, so the calm levelling effects of tranquil scenes from nature that would counteract the intense and fragmented elements of Victor's and Penelope's lives, were not appropriate for Karen. She was already grounded and showing all the signs of real Kapha slowness. She worked in thoroughly professional but absolutely dull conditions and in un-coordinated cacophony at home. Her Kapha solidity has become too static and the earth and water elements that define Kapha types had become, to all intents and purposes, as sticky as mud. Karen needed some fire bringing into her life to burn away the complacency she knew she had succumbed to. She didn't need to turn away from nature and her appreciation of seascapes could form the basis for new experiences.

Of the three of them Karen would benefit most from wild, stormy conditions and from the sight of elemental natural forces in their full power. Surfing beaches, breaking waves, stormy mountain scenes and vigorous walks over wild craggy ridges on blustery changeable days would be ideal ways for Karen to get the exercise she needed in surroundings that would be visually stimulating. Rough seas, vigorous activity and movement and contrast were all good for her, better in fact than those settled, soothing sights she'd been used to. What was interesting was the way that Karen would process the apparent chaos and disorder of nature through her eyes and mind. There is an incipient anarchy about the wild places that would enliven Karen's earthy stability. Her Kapha qualities of smoothness, with slow structured movement, would be balanced by these unbridled experiences. Using the analogy of a camera viewfinder, by looking at such scenes and activities Karen would bring a Golden Section of her own inner order to frame the excitement and random forces she saw.

Karen's holidays and activities took her away from many potentially energising sources and Linda showed her how lively street life in all its forms would be great for shifting her Kapha slowness. The careless scatter of street signs and graphics, markets, western malls and eastern bazaars and those kinds of high octane settings were exactly what her Kapha eyes needed. Once again, she would process these chaotic sights with her Kapha stability. The sight and sensation of life pulsating in crowded thoroughfares would be like a shot in the arm. Jaded eyes would be invigorated by the variety and energy of it all. She might not participate in a whole new set of activities, but being present, watching and entering into the spirit of these events would be good for her. Hotel suites might be the good life for some, but vibrant, pulsating street life was what Karen needed most. Her home and her wardrobe needed to retain some of the visual drama she had unwittingly created balanced by co-ordination and restraint. Bold contrasts and colourful accents was the theme Linda introduced to Karen's colour schemes.

Chapter 4

The Senses:
Hearing, Touch and Spirit

———————————

All of the new knowledge they were accumulating was central to our trio's renewal, but they needed to take daily action to sustain the changes through their senses. Most of us are fortunate to have the six senses of sound, touch, sight, taste, smell and spirit. Like most people, Victor, Penelope and Karen only used some of them for some of the time, yet these senses are our greatest resource. Victor had spent hours and hours in the gym training his body but hardly any time on the rest of himself. Penelope had an important job, was very active physically and socially, but was failing to understand her own needs. Karen had most ingredients for a happy life but wasn't facing up to her own habits of procrastination and her tendency to live behind a protective shell. Linda now showed them how more small daily acts would develop their senses and intuition to make the best of all their resources.

Like many people, Victor took for granted a great deal of what went on around him and neglected himself badly. He thought he was doing well, and he spent enough money on entertainment, the gym and clothes, but he hadn't been choosing experiences that would suit his Vata type because he hadn't known about it before. Instead he allowed media, friends and family to influence his choice of sensory experience. What Victor was about to learn was how little attention he had really paid to himself and his surroundings and what great opportunities existed for feeling alive and happy in his own Vata body.

At first Penelope "needed no help in getting in touch with herself" and she'd spent a lot of time pursuing healthy interests and yet she was forced to acknowledge that she was too often stressed and angry and actually spent little time being reflective and quiet. Her drive and determination usually had her fired up and active, which was an asset in her professional life, but she spent very little time away from high energy situations and even her ways of relaxing were intense. If one word could summarise her general experience of life it would be "heated"—physically and emotionally. She had been used to controlling most aspects of her life and could see that she needed to create opportunities for letting go and absorbing softer experiences into her life.

Karen had begun to mistake complacency for comfort and after talking to Linda she began to see that she had spent years in increasing levels of inactivity. There was a distinct pattern to the way she had dealt with crises and changes generally and it involved avoiding a pro-active response and settling for managing the least-worst option. There had been many times when she'd avoided problems at work rather than deal with them as they occurred. She avoided arguments like the plague when, in fact, there had been a number of instances with colleagues and her family when conflicts had needed to be aired, to be brought out into the open, that would have run the risk of challenging confrontations. There had also been many occasions when she'd wished her friend would go for a different kind of holiday, but she never pushed her ideas forward. She was completely stuck and she knew it.

They looked at the sense of hearing

Sound is energy made audible. When an object makes a noise, it sends vibrations (sound waves) speeding through the air. These vibrations are then funneled into our ear canals by the outer ear. As the vibrations move into our middle ear, they hit our eardrum and cause it to vibrate as well. This sets off a chain reaction of vibrations that are eventually interpreted by our brains. We literally feel the vibrationary quality of sound with our whole being and have an amazing ability to respond to a wide dynamic range of auditory input.

Sounds have the capacity to move us to tears, to send us to war and to nurture and comfort us. Sound soothes our troubles and excites our senses at a visceral level. It heals us and it can damage us. We absorb the sequences and gradations of musical scales and modalities and the abstract structures of many musical forms, and we conjure up from memory the most complex patterns and rhythms of notes that carry emotional force and lift our spirits. We express ideas through the subtleties and nuances of sounds and savour the richness of words through poetry and prose. Sound conveys threat and alarm, tenderness and love, verbally and non-verbally. Sounds, like smell, are powerfully linked to memory; a lullaby or a cherished song connects us immediately to a source that may be many years distant, with absolute clarity. We can't see, hold, smell or touch sounds but they have long enduring effects on our quality of life. Within Ayurveda sound is a fundamental healing tool and through our sense of hearing we connect with every life form and with our past memories. We do this by consciously experiencing the sound of running water and rain, leaves rustling, birdsong and the range of life that exists outside our heads and we use chants and mantras with the potential to create profound change at a cellular level within our bodies. Science is beginning to recognise what Ayurvedic seers knew thousands of years ago; existence is a vibrationary phenomenon and our daily experience of sound should be something that re-charges our batteries and helps to renew and rebuild our cells. We are natural beings and we need auditory experiences that strengthen our connection with each other and with nature, in the same way that plants needs sunlight. Our sensory memory needs refreshing in the same way our thirst needs to be satisfied; and this refreshment comes from the conscious application of healing sound.

Our bodies are miracles of design and our ability to hear comes as a result of some remarkable engineering that even now, with our high tech 21st century skills, we could not replicate efficiently at anything like the tiny scale of the human ear. Even today with the most sophisticated development of computers and electronic digital equipment it would be impossible to duplicate the function of the inner ear in a machine even as large as a refrigerator. However, the inner ear (only the size of a pea) is capable of processing a whole range of sound.

Sound waves generated by mechanical forces cause the eardrum—and, in turn, the three tiny bones of the middle ear—to vibrate. The last of these three bones (the stapes, or "stirrup") jiggles a flexible layer of tissue at the base of the cochlea. This pressure sends waves rippling along the basilar membrane, stimulating some of its hair cells. These hair cells are so sensitive that deflecting the tip of a bundle of hair cells by the width of an atom is enough to make the cell respond. This infinitesimal movement, which might be caused by a very low, quiet sound at the threshold of hearing, is equivalent to displacing the top of the Eiffel Tower by only half an inch.

The basilar membrane then sends out a rapid-fire code of electrical signals that communicate the frequency, intensity, and duration of a sound. The messages finally reach the auditory areas of the cerebral cortex within the brain, which processes and interprets these signals as a musical phrase, a dripping faucet, a human voice, or any of the thousands of sounds in the world around us at any particular moment. Our auditory systems are remarkably efficient and sensitive. They can distinguish between a whisper and an explosion, between the differing qualities of sound within a certain frequency and they can protect themselves from the effects of extreme ranges of sound.

The hair cells' response is amazingly rapid. In order to be able to process sounds at the highest frequency range of human hearing, hair cells must be able to turn current on and off 20,000 times per second. They are capable of even more astonishing speeds in bats and whales, which can distinguish sounds at frequencies as high as 200,000 cycles per second. Photoreceptors in the eye are much slower. The visual system is so slow that when you look at a movie at 24 frames per second, it seems continuous, without any flicker. Contrast 24 frames per second with 20,000 cycles per second. The auditory system is a thousand times faster.

These comparisons between the relative efficiency of the ear and the eye have been made by scientists at the Howard Hughes Medical Centre in the USA and they reveal the extent to which we take the gift of hearing for granted and how little we use the uniquely dynamic capability of this powerful sense.

Cycles and frequencies mean little to the layperson, but more anecdotal descriptions of these qualities are useful. Researchers found that if the eye was forced to demonstrate the same capacity for perception as the ear and distinguish the tremendous difference between the sound of a cannon and a whisper, it is likely that the eye would have to be protected externally. Fortunately for us, the ear protects itself with built in mechanisms. The auditory system is able to distinguish efficiently sound as low as 20 cycles/sec. (hertz = Hz), and as high as 20,000 Hz. Physically processing such a wide range of frequencies constitutes a truly miraculous perfection of engineering. If the eyes were exposed to the same extremes it would be the equivalent of looking directly into bright sunlight. After such an experience the individual would have to wait a few minutes before being able to focus the eyes completely. Nonetheless, the ear can switch between the whisper and the cannon sound with little or no effort. We can filter out unwanted sounds and consciously or unconsciously select what we choose to hear. We can live close to roads and learn to ignore the sound of traffic but still hear the faint sound of a child crying or a tap dripping. In a crowded restaurant we can shut out extraneous chatter and concentrate on the person whispering confidences to us across the table.

Sound mediates the way we communicate. Cacophony creates cacophony, turmoil ferments further turmoil and, whilst variety enriches our experience of life, there has been an escalation in the damaging levels of sound that we are exposed to nowadays. This is not simply reactionary fuddy-duddy opinion but an observation based on the evidence of increased population levels, changes in social behaviour and recreational trends. More people, more traffic, and more pressure lead to more noise. This is a simple statement of fact. Our workplace and our homes are the places where we can balance these increased levels of noise. Just as we may rest our eyes by gazing into the distance and by looking at soothing greens and blues, we need to relieve our hearing mechanism with different qualities of sound. We have physical needs within this realm of sound that correspond with our physical need to eat and drink and sleep. We need the corrective frequencies of good quality sound.

Everyone needs to experience these sounds as often as possible, preferably on a daily basis: rustling leaves; wind chimes; repetitive natural sounds that soothe like a mantra, such as rainfall, waves, streams and waterfalls; a range of musical styles; solo instruments and ensemble music; songs and lullabies; and the natural domestic sounds made whilst cooking. These vibrations retune our auditory sense and our soul. They heal damaged bodies and our immune system. They take us back to ourselves.

It is vital that we nurture our senses and sustain them into advancing old age. The delicate hair cells deep within our ears are susceptible to damage from sustained exposure to loud noise, also to heredity factors and illness. Since the beginning of industrialization our way of life has involved ever increasing decibel levels and now many other causes of excessive noise, such as mobile phones and iPods, all contribute to our levels of auditory saturation. A sad statistic is that people tend to lose 40% of their ear's hair cells by the age of 65. Once destroyed, these cells do not regenerate. The time to look after our senses is now. We know that a diet of takeaway food and sugary drinks leads to obesity and ill-health. We wouldn't dream of following such a regime on a sustained basis. By the same token we should modulate our auditory intake and give ourselves the best sounds we can hear. The nature of what is best for us varies according to our dosha and our state of balance at any time, but those soothing sounds such as described above, are core requirements for everyone.

Hearing for a Vata person: Victor worked in a media office that was a hive of activity. There was always a background noise and it was usually frenetic. Victor was a devotee of clubs and all the heavy sounds that went with them, and he had CDs in his car and others he played at home, all with the same kind of driving bass and rhythms. It had become a habit to play the stuff but the more Linda talked to him the more he realised that this music actually aggravated him when he wasn't on the dance floor. He learned that soothing natural sounds that might not be great for the clubs, would have a powerful grounding effect on his Vata brain. This was really important because sounds and music that rooted Victor in the natural would have a great levelling effect on his disorganised and hyperactive mind. He discovered that classical music at home helped greatly in bringing him peace and clarity, and he actually began to enjoy the depth of stillness and quietness he was able to experience. It was also vital that he listened to the sounds he made when cooking, to expand the sensory experience of eating.

...and to a Pitta person. Penelope was similar to Victor in that her working environment was quite noisy and challenging, even when things were going well. She had placed herself on the firing line as a result of her early promotion; and being an agent of change in such a high profile position, with her daily menu of teaching, meetings and difficult interactions, created levels and qualities of sound that were really quite antagonistic. Driving dance rhythms in the clubs and soundtracks to aerobics added to a generally low quality of auditory experience. Talking to Linda helped Penelope realise that she was actually starving herself of soothing natural sounds. She spent little time in nature for the sake of relaxation, where activity could have been combined with hearing the silence and the sounds of wind and water all of which was vital to restore her Pitta balance. She loved the music she heard in Morocco and other countries, with haunting chants and religious prayers and mantras sung to slower pulsing rhythms, and she got goose bumps from hearing many kinds of classical music; yet she had separated these sounds from everyday life. She learned that they enabled her to find a calm centre that placed her heavy workload into context as soon as she heard them. She began to feel calmer at home, thus easing the tensions with her boyfriend. Like Victor, cooking sounds were important in helping her regain an earthy grounded quality.

   ...and to a Kapha person. Karen was completely different from both Victor and Penelope. Her home and working environment were quiet and she ensured that stress was kept at bay by ignoring it at source level. Her office life involved low levels of sound; music wasn't allowed and any conversation was low-key and quite technical in content—apart from the odd bit of friendly chat. Her social life also had little by way of stimulating sound or music. The Yoga classes where the teacher used a beautiful but very calm soundtrack, the hotel breaks and other holidays were all great experiences, but involved only low-key or natural sounds. Karen loved natural sounds and they are indeed good for everyone's sense of connection with nature; however listening to Linda, Karen realised she had absolutely no peaks and troughs of auditory stimulation. Every sound she experienced was low and harmonious and her natural Kapha steadiness already contained this quality. She actually needed stimulation, not sedation, and lively music such as rock and roll, salsa and similar sounds that she could also dance to were exactly what were required. Linda showed her that sound would lift her whole level of energy and help begin a process of change. Karen already had calmness in her life, but that, combined with her Kapha tendency to lethargy had subdued the fire in her belly. They both agreed on the recipe for igniting that fire.

They looked at the sense of touch

The sense of touch is of such importance that infants of all species die without it. So do adults, but more slowly. The sense of touch occurs primarily through our skin and we sense touch with our whole bodies whereas the senses of sight, hearing, smell, and taste are located in specific parts of the body. Touch is our oldest, most primitive sense. It's the first sense we experience in the womb and the last one we lose before death. As infants our early experiences occur through touch and we learn to assess our surroundings through our skin, which protects us as we feel our way around, sampling the differences between a soft blanket and a hard wood floor. As adults we communicate tenderness and love, tension and rage to each other through touch. We caress with incredible lightness and hammer with explosive power. Within the Arts we have a remarkable capacity to express ourselves creatively and touch is a primary healing modality for many holistic disciplines. The fine degress of control we have over our senses of touch is a common factor in all these experiences.

We feel touch throughout every square centimetre of our bodies. We have about twenty different types of nerve endings that all send messages to our brains and they are located all over our bodies with about 100 touch receptors in each of our fingertips alone, making them especially sensitive. The most common receptors are for heat, cold, pain, and pressure or touch. Pain receptors warn us of potentially damaging conditions and in addition to pain, the touch system allows for a variety of sensations including vibration, pressure, stretch, itch, texture, and temperature and humidity. The system is sensitive to certain chemical states like painful tissue acidity, the result of inflammation or infection. Touch also underlies the brain's sense of where parts of the body are positioned at any given moment, crucial to motor control. Touch takes many forms. Through our touch system we are able to differentiate between fleeting touch and heavier and more sustained pressure, which may ultimately lead to us taking protective measures. Light touch allows us to detect fleeting sensations such as an insect landing on our arm. If the insect remains there, we lose sensitivity to it and if we look away we don't even feel it.

Some areas of the body are more sensitive than others because they have more nerve endings. Anyone who has ever bitten their own tongue will know about the number of nerve endings in this particular organ. The sides of our tongues have a lot of nerve endings that are very sensitive to pain but the tongue is not as good at sensing hot or cold, which is why it is easy to burn our mouths when we eat something really hot. Our fingertips are also very sensitive and blind people use their fingertips to read Braille by feeling the patterns of raised dots on paper.

Skin weighs from six to ten pounds in an adult and is made of three layers: the epidermis or the top layer, the dermis or middle layer and the subcutis, the lower layer which contains insulating fat and muscle. The epidermis is about as thick as a piece of paper and serves as a shield against the elements. Here, over the course of a few weeks, new cells are created which migrate to the skin's surface, die, and are then shed to form the dust that permeates our living spaces. The epidermis, which is waterproof, also contains the cells that produce melanin, the agent responsible for skin colour. These cells on the outside surface of the skin are dead because cells in the lower part of the epidermis are constantly multiplying, pushing cells upward as more are made. We lose between 30,000 and 40,000 skin cells every minute (up to 9 lbs. of skin cells every year), but our skin does not wear away because it constantly renews itself, fortunately for us. In fact it is beneficial for us to assist the natural process of skin renewal through exfoliation (removing dead skin) and protecting the new layer with appropriate oils and creams.

Below the epidermis is the dermis, home to the proteins collagen and elastin, which ensure that we recover our shape after it's been pushed and pinched. The dermis is responsible for our sense of touch, and is filled with tiny nerve endings which collect information about the things our bodies come in contact with. They carry this information to the spinal cord, which sends messages to the brain. Our brains assemble an overall "touch picture" from nerve signals, and we might describe certain aspects of this touch picture with words such as hot or cold, dry or moist, smooth or rough. We have about 50 touch receptors for every square centimeter of skin and about 5 million sensory cells overall. The dermis is packed with a dense network of blood vessels that nourish the skin and help maintain body temperature by constricting and dilating in response to cold and heat.

Finally, below the dermis is the subcutis, which contains fat and muscle that insulate the internal organs and act as an energy reservoir for the body. During pregnancy most of the organs develop early on, but in a foetus the process of skin-building takes the entire pre-birth cycle.

A layer of skin, usually only about 5 mm thick, is the only protection that the insides of our body have against the range of environmental factors all around us. It protects us from harmful things such as bacteria. It keeps the water in our bodies from drying up because it has a waterproof epidermis. Oil glands in the dermis produce oils that help keep the skin moist. The dermis also regulates the temperature of our bodies because layers of fat help keep us warm whilst sweat glands let the body give off moisture through the skin, helping to cool us.

Fortunately this barrier we call skin translates into the power of touch. Touch has an amazing power for infants. There is ample evidence to show that an infant that goes untouched often dies; studies show that infants who are rarely touched have brains 20% smaller than those who are touched a lot. Infants need to be touched and comforted and the quality of touch is important, especially with softness and sensitivity. Children who are picked up, cuddled, cradled, rocked, petted, and stroked have been shown to gain weight and grow faster and to start crawling, walking, and grabbing earlier. They are also more alert and active, sleep more soundly, develop stronger immune systems and have higher IQs than those left alone in their cribs without being touched. Newborns especially love the touch of others, mostly their parents; they love to be stroked and massaging a baby is so beneficial that it's now a common therapeutic technique in many neonatal intensive care units.

It is believed that the reason babies crave touch may be because they have grown accustomed to the constant sensations of the fluid filled womb. Swaddling in snug blankets may replace that constant stimulation, and also prevent the startling sensation of movement from uncoordinated arms and legs. Warm baths fulfill the same need.

There is so much evidence for the benefits of touch to babies that we can simply accept what common sense tells us. Humans thrive as a result of benign, caring tactile experiences and research has shown that touch may be as important to a baby's physical, emotional, and cognitive development as eating and sleeping. In a Harvard Medical School study of an overcrowded orphanage in Romania, researchers found that babies who lay for hours without physical human contact suffered stunted growth and had abnormal levels of cortisol. All of the growth and developmental factors apply to animals as well as humans.

This need to touch and be touched does not change as we reach adulthood, but unfortunately most people's experience of a range of touch sensations reduces rather than grows. With so much common sense and scientific evidence to validate the importance of touch between humans, it is sad to acknowledge that social conventions in 21st Century western society place constraints on the ways in which adults communicate through this most fundamental mode of expression. Teachers can no longer touch children in the way a caring adult was once able to do and doctors are forced to achieve targets that preclude time and touch with their patients. Artificial barriers have been created through fear of litigation and lack of faith, depriving children and adults of essential, grounding experiences. That fear translates into separation, mistrust and to an inability to express ourselves fully. Ritualised contact, such as handshaking, backslapping and hugging are merely vestiges of a greater component of human communication. They demonstrate the limits that have gradually been imposed on the physical range of expression we are capable of. We believe that "high fives," punching the air and triumphant clenched fist waving are inadequate alternatives to more meaningful contact. We use the expression "giving strokes" as an analogy to describe the act of praising someone rather than actually giving the physical strokes that communicate more directly and which are truly needed.

Sadly, we have become inhibited about touching to the extent of being touch-illiterate. Adults, especially parents, desperately need to learn about touch for themselves in order to foster self-confidence and awareness in their children. Jim once worked with a teenage girl whose experience of life could only allow her to communicate affection through hard punching and strong physical interaction. She had never known gentleness and didn't have the ability to express tenderness other than through what was, effectively, a form of aggression. She was lively and cheeky but had a protective shell, which manifested as toughness and "friendly" punches that deadened the arm of any recipient. The more affectionate she wanted to be, the more frequent the punches. She had not experienced a full range of touch in non-threatening circumstances and didn't know how to express herself. Hers is an extreme example, but in recent years most people have become inhibited about touch.

Each sense contributes to the whole self and sharpening one sense boosts our receptivity to the others. Self-awareness grows incrementally through exercise, in the same way that muscles and endurance grow through training. Touching objects strengthens our knowledge and awareness of the external world. Touching ourselves strengthens our sense of self. Dislocation and disassociation occur when we don't touch. Connecting with life and objects outside ourselves reinforces our relationship to the environment, to cellular memories and to sensory factors that enlarge us. We grow through contact in exactly the same way that babies become stronger and healthier as a result of nurturing touch and broader tactile experiences. At the quantum level every living thing is composed of the five elements. We build our bodies by eating these elements, and we strengthen our senses through direct contact with the same elements.

The sense of touch is in direct alignment with the heart chakra and is probably the most important connection to our emotions. From touch we develop self-love, comfort and compassion. Our other senses do not connect so directly with our feelings but from touch we strengthen awareness of our place in the world, in our surroundings and immediate environment, experiencing nurturance without intellectual filters. This is a critical point. Sensuality and the pleasures of touch create strong healthy babies and strengthen our adult sensibility. Touch bypasses the barrage of sound, vision and structure that surrounds us and it connects us to elemental feelings. If as children, or as adults on a path to growth and enlightenment, we only receive a limited range of touch stimuli we are limited; as children, if we only heard people shouting at each other we would grow up shouting ourselves; if all we saw around us was running and fighting, we would run and fight. Unless we have direct experience of the range of human expression we limit our own potential. So it is with touch and, unfortunately, limitation is the norm for large sections of society. We have become accustomed to the extremes in most things and touch is no exception. Tactile experiences are too hard, too soft, red hot or freezing and subtlety is hidden away in danger of being lost. Commercial exteriors and interiors are designed to manipulate our senses and move us on to the next retail opportunity, and although these may seem like generalisations, they are true for the broader categories of everyday life. Commercially speaking, subtlety is an exclusive domain, often pushed into the background, yet vital for our well-being. Practice sharpens our senses and our level of brain activity and we need to experience the full range of tactile experiences to avoid limiting our expectations.

Most adults have learned to compartmentalise touch. They withhold from social touch and create barriers that limit communication and which require great linguistic endeavor to replace what they have forgotten how to do in other ways. Sensuality, nurturing touch and knowledge of the self are confused with sexuality. People have lost confidence in their ability to touch themselves and others without sexual intent and this creates isolation. Adults recoil from social touch because they have reduced touch solely to the realm of sexuality. For many people the only time they have tactile experiences is within sexual intercourse, but because of the constraints they have placed upon the way they touch even those experiences are limited. In sex therapy couples are taught to touch each other gently on safe areas of the body (arms, legs, torsos, not the genitals) to build awareness of themselves and each other. People who suffer blockages (often known, unpleasantly, as "frigidity") are taught, under therapy to self-examine their bodies, to learn self-massage and become familiar with their skin so as to build confidence, enabling them to move out of the sexuality trap. Sensuality is a rich gift that has a context. Our physical body is the vehicle for the best, most varied and the richest range of sensory activity that we can create. Touch crosses time, gender and age boundaries and makes us human. We simply have to re-learn how to enjoy this sense.

Linda introduced Victor, Penelope and Karen to some activities that would be good for all three doshas. They all needed to shake up their appreciation of touch. Until they are challenged, most people cut themselves off from their sense of touch and it takes conscious effort to feel again. Touch takes time; the sight of texture is also important, since we can feel smoothness and roughness with our eyes as well as our hands. We can see the subtle nap of suede or the sheen of silk, and the sense of sight compliments touch in many contexts.

Becoming a parent re-awakens our ability to respond in a tactile way. Holding and cuddling a child is probably the most powerful tactile experience we will ever have, and though none of our three subjects were quite ready to have babies yet, Karen did get to snuggle up to her younger nieces and nephews occasionally. Pet therapy is a good way to re-establish touch, by feeling the grain and texture of hair and the muscle of other living creatures. Linda wasn't suggesting they should all go out and buy a dog, but lots of other opportunities existed. Horse riding or trekking is an accessible way of coming into contact with vibrant creatures possessing power and grace, something that all three of them could consider. Animal sanctuaries, zoos and friends with pets provided other opportunities. They needed to remain open to the moments when they could, safely, see, touch and feel cats, dogs, birds, horses, cows and other animals. People who own pets are known to suffer less from stress, and our three subjects could top up their stress-resistance banks.

Baking improves the sense of touch; kneading dough and rolling pastry combines large and small-scale movement and requires muscle and finesse in equal measure. Baking strikes a powerfully earthy cord, perfect for Vata and Pitta types and requires enough effort to offset any excessively heavy Kapha tendencies. It obviously fits in well with all the other forms of food preparation too, but there is a spirituality that comes from working with our most basic food source that benefits everyone.

Later Linda took them back to the park where they had worked with smell. She wanted them to note every detail of an everyday sensual experience. It was a warm day and they felt the heat on their faces when they faced the sun. Linda got them to take off their shoes. They felt the rough texture of paving stones underfoot and walked down sharp edged steps. They felt each step's hardness as they went down, gripping a handrail that was polished and smooth through the passage of thousands of hands. The metal was warm to the touch and was attached to the boundary wall every half-metre by a bulbous bracket that bumped their hands as they slid down the rail. They got to a gravelly level with twigs and small sharp stones, then moved on to softer ground where grass swallowed their feet, covering them in clinging dampness. They walked around for some time feeling the coolness evaporating from the wet grass and then eventually put on their shoes again.

There was nothing unusual about this particular experience and yet there was something very special about it because they had consciously chosen to examine with intent a small microcosm of the world, with hundreds of fleeting impressions that they so easily took for granted. They began to understand Linda's point. Life is full of sensations and possibilities and as children each one is an adventure, but by the time we reach adulthood we have become blasé about the ordinary. Attention to the details creates magic that enrichens our lives. As with Proust's realisation of the connection between smell and memory, all moments that contain precise sensations (often experienced through physical activity), become saturated with impressions that make us grow.

With touch we can prepare ourselves by asking some simple questions. Is this surface hot or cold, cool or warm? Is it rough or smooth, polished or matt? Does my skin slide along it or drag? Is it made up of many pieces or is it larger and more continuous? What do my fingers feel after I've touched it? Does it remind me of other surfaces? These and other questions help to raise our expectations in the same way that the smell of food enhances its taste. If there are any doubts about how to open up to touch on this basis, watching a child's sensitivity to new tactile sensations provides a great lesson in awareness.

So Linda looked at touch and what that meant to a Vata person. Victor hadn't really thought about touch, but immediately he recognised that the dry skin he'd often suffered from affected the way he experienced textures. Linda introduced him to oils that would ease this dryness and which was the first stage in preparing for touch. She showed him how to self-massage and how to massage his girlfriend. She stressed that his Vata body needed slow, firm, nurturing touch, not the vigorous heavy massage that many people opt for and Victor learned that sandalwood oil was great for him for both for its oily qualities and its smell, as was frankincense and sesame oil. He could learn to soak for relaxation rather than his usual habit of diving in and out of the shower, using those same oils. A keener sense of touch would strengthen the grounding effect he was working for. One way could be through clothing, and wools and fleeces are great for nurturing Vatas. Victor never wore hats normally and that was another simple change that would improve his sense of being nurtured.

He would be able to ground his airy Vata personality even more by taking opportunities to touch new and unfamiliar surfaces from natural elements around him such as rocks, trees, water, furnishings and fabrics in his home and at work and also the built environment. Although it had never even occurred to him before, gardening would be a great activity for Victor to look into, and while he lived in a flat, by introducing potted plants, indoor "window boxes" and an indoor herb garden he could bring the earth into his home interior. Victor was fortunate in that there were some beautifully tended council gardens not too far away, as well as a stately home with spectacular landscape architecture, trees and terraced gardens full of a fantastic variety of plants, flowers and shrubs that were both soothing and stimulating enough for anyone. These places provided an oasis for his Vata needs.

Lastly, the texture and feel of his food would extend Victor's tactile range and Linda talked through the need for him to slow down his methods of preparation to savour not only the taste and smell, but also the texture of each raw ingredient.

...and to a Pitta person. Penelope's general experiences of touch involved little in the way of sensitivity. Her badminton and aerobics, dancing and domestic life all involved vigorous physical sensations one way or another, and holidays and social life were conducted at a fast pace and with an overall heartiness and vigour that were anything but sensitive. Linda showed Penelope how her Pitta vigour needed balancing with sensitive, slow and caring touch sensations. Self-massage was important and also quiet time with her boyfriend could introduce this quality directly into her daily routines, using lavender essential oil and cooling coconut oil that were for her body type. There was a Jacuzzi at the health club that would give her a great tactile experience, and Linda suggested that Penelope should include swimming into her activities, since Pitta types are really soothed by what is essentially a sensual cooling and fluid form of activity. Beach life was recommended for her, but not in the heat of the sun, and whether by the sea or along lakeside walks, the feel of sand underfoot, water close by and cooling shade would be a soothing tonic. Images and sounds of the sea at home and work would complete the healing effect. Penelope had a small garden and Linda urged her to spend time planning and designing a new layout that included herbs, shrubs and larger plants that would ground Penelope's fiery personality and provide something she could share with her boyfriend. Digging and shifting soil would be great exercise for them both. She could plan a mediation space within the garden and Linda showed her how a garden theme could be developed in the house so that outside and inside environments could be linked, practically and in spirit.

Penelope's Pitta temperament, skin and body temperature would all benefit from finer fabrics than she had been wearing, cotton and linen being excellent for Pittas, and her home would be much better for the introduction of natural fabrics and textures. She needed to be able to breathe through her skin and relieve her natural heat, so the easy-care fabrics she'd been wearing needed revising to include natural fibres. Penelope's Pitta fire needed gentle cooling and increasing sensitivity through her sense of touch, through contact with natural elements and textures, through the texture of her food and through a general slowing down of her pace that she would gain as she responded to these new tactile sensations. This would lead to balance.

....and to a Kapha person. Karen's quiet life, quiet job and quiet holidays had all reduced her sensory input to a low level. The only physical activity she undertook, Yoga, was conducted in an atmosphere of religious calm and she actually had few strong physical sensations in any area of her life. Karen didn't need a lot of convincing when Linda pointed out what was missing from her tactile experiences and it was obvious that her Kapha solidity and stability needed stimulating in a big way. Of all the doshas, Kapha needs vigorous touch and can withstand heavy exercise. Karen could take up the massage options in those hotel spas she went to, and learn how to self-massage with relatively quick and very firm touch and technique, using citrus or spicy oils to add zest. She had a garden but paid a gardener to do the work once a month or more often in the summer. Linda put a stop to this arrangement, as Karen had the strength to undertake some fairly heavy work on her own behalf, shifting things around and establishing some new features, all of which would build Karen's bodily awareness. There was a good opportunity to set up lighting features that would add rich texture to her view outside at night. Linda suggested bringing some Japanese elements into the outside spaces, with stones and fine gravel to create crunchy textures and sounds that would be perfect for stimulating Karen's senses.

To balance her life, Karen needed to add fast movement and dancing would be a great way for her natural Kapha grace to combine with the sense of touch and rhythm to boost her metabolism and spirits. Her country walks provided one opportunity to break into more adventurous distances and locations, with gorge walking, ridge walking and scrambling on the revised agenda. Urban locations with their particular textures ranging from chrome to the coarsest building materials were also excellent for energising her Kapha temperament, combined with walks through city streets, feeling her own pace and the bustle of other people brushing by. She needed to find pavement cafes and similarly lively settings and new urban sensations. Even the bookshop that she visited had lots of stimulating contrasts between the bookishness and the urbanity of the people passing through. New coarser textures in her domestic surroundings and her wardrobe would also help to reinvigorate her dormant tactile senses.

They looked at the sense of spirit

Spirit is the factor that links all our senses. When we approach our full potential we are whole both as individuals and collectively as a species. Our minds and bodies are connected, they function harmoniously and we regain contact with a universal sense of spirit that we reach through practical activities with our other senses (many of which have been outlined already), and through paying attention to the gift of life. In the world of form, our Mother Earth is tangible to us through the senses, and we have touched upon the role that each separate sense plays in expanding our perception and our potential. The integration of our experiences and receptivity to spirit, to our inner vibration raises our awareness beyond the level of the mundane, the neglectful and the destructive.

The essence of life lies within every cell of our bodies. We take in the five elements through nutrition and through our senses, but the sense of spirit resides within every cell, in the element of ether, with all the potential for past, present and future that the great sages described so many centuries ago. Through ether we connect with the life force of every living thing. In quantum terms we are vibratory creations, and apparent differences between life forms and all "solid" matter are illusory at the most microscopic level. These quantum level vibrations occur within the element of ether. Our vibrationary core might appear to be inaccessible until we feel our reaction to mantra, chanting and to primordial sound. At these times we leave mind-dominance behind and enter heightened consciousness where we experience the inspirational properties of space, where interiors and exteriors shift our perception, and we are struck by natural beauty, by childlike innocence and the natural grace in humans or animals. At these moments we communicate directly though our sense of spirit and our reactions are unfiltered by intellectual considerations. These are the times when we experience our true potential and we connect to what we observe at the deepest level. It is possible to seek out these moments and stay within that level of awareness when we find it. Every such experience expands our capacity to feel, to be human and, most critically, to be part of the natural living organism that is our planet. Developing our senses through the activities we have described cements and integrates our complete cellular self to the wholeness of all other life on earth. Every single time we have these experiences we rebuild ourselves.

That is why we work with our spiritual attributes. They are the least tangible and yet the most essential of all our gifts. We are blessed with the ability to communicate in many different ways, and we have the resources to do so across continents and oceans. These gifts are not incidental; they are not inconsequential. We can speak and feel through our minds, through our bodies and through a power that is infinitely greater than anything we can invent or construct. We are the sum of all our experiences and we are connected to all around us. We have marvellous gifts, including six senses with which to experience the incredible richness and variety of life. If we don't strive to reach our full potential, if we don't feel our full emotional and sensory range, then we waste the time we've been given here on this earth.

We have an obligation to our children and grandchildren to nurture them within an environment that provides for their needs. Our planet and its ecosystems are the physical manifestations of how we value and regard life. In this respect we are what we do, not what we say and we have been systematically consuming our precious planet for hundreds of years while putting nothing back to replenish that which sustains us. Global warming is a terrible reality; species are being wiped out; rainforests that oxygenate the planet continue to be depleted and at every level, from government downwards, hardly anything is being done to counteract the global scale of the damage. At a local level, economic growth and speculation lead to building sites that obliterate local habitats. The population shift towards cities means that young and old alike have fewer opportunities to experience nature at first hand and they can only learn from secondary sources such as the web, which highlights a 21st Century dilemma. We think we are clever; we have access to possessions on a previously unimaginable scale and we have begun to equate this with joy.

However, possessions don't fill the spiritual emptiness that has insinuated itself into the lives of millions. Poverty of spirit and loss of community are like a disease and until we rediscover our role in the natural cycles of life we will not halt our progress towards spiritual and physical desolation. We have the universe within us. We are nature. We are the environment, not a super race that grazes from it. Everything that we do to others we do to ourselves. Enlightened leaders and philosophers have spoken these words for thousands of years and perhaps now, because scientists are saying the same thing, we will listen. It is only by honouring our role within the wider universe, by breaking free from a collective egocentricity and by seeing the power of the mind (and its capacity for invention in a different context) as a tool that can contribute to existence and not dominate it, that we will survive and grow spiritually. As individuals we can begin to make a difference, because change creates bigger change, but we have to start now, before it's too late. What we do to ourselves affects the wider environment; the outside is a reflection of the inside. Spiritual growth comes from practical activity and awareness and first hand contact with the natural world is a pre-requisite for health. In pragmatic terms we begin by working on ourselves and on our children; we work with our physical and emotional debris, and thus create health and awareness from within.

Victor, Penelope and Karen had each created lives within environments that they believed to be healthy and conducive to happiness, but like most people their ideas and beliefs were founded on media-influenced or generalist principles that paid no attention to the subtle variations that occur within body types or to the greater spiritual dimension of life. It was surprising to them the extent to which what was good for one was bad for another, yet working through a structured process with Linda they learned how to understand themselves in ways they hadn't imagined. They learned to recognise inherent traits and tendencies for what they were and not see them as faults, but as aspects of themselves that could be creative and useful, and which could be balanced through changes to nutrition, activity and environment. They learned to step outside their emotional condition and see themselves differently, not as victims of their surroundings but as people with the power of choice. Most importantly they learned how to pay attention to what was going on inside themselves and how to respond creatively.

The sense of spirit for a Vata person. This was the big one for Victor. As soon as that word cropped up he leapt to the "religious" conclusion that so many people do, but Linda explained that our sense of spirit meant something much different. Victor needed to reinforce his connection with something greater than the surface details of life that went on around him. Most of us do but different dosha types need it in different ways. We all benefit from the realisation that there is something "bigger than us" and we can find that in the grandest of settings and also the humblest. Victor's greatest need was for mental stillness to quieten his changeable Vata mind. For that he needed to consciously stop himself for a short while several times everyday. Peace and stillness can be found in two ways; from our surroundings and from inside ourselves. Victor would gain a lot by visiting great architectural spaces such as cathedrals, churches, etc., for the calming effect of their structural integrity and their intent, planning and design; he would gain a lot by walking in the country and by the sea; most importantly he would gain by daily meditation. Linda taught Victor some simple meditation techniques that would bring about big changes. Meditation is the best way to "stop the mind" and Victor could begin the sanity-saving process with short periods of daily mediation that would bring peace and strength.

...and for a Pitta person. Penelope urgently needed calmness and a change to the hothouse life she had created. Whilst Pitta people are not airy and changeable like Vatas, they still require the same quality of mental stillness and a release from the driven state they take themselves into. Penelope's authoritative role in work, her competitive nature and her demanding social round all took her away from her spiritual core. She rarely reflected on things that weren't governed by professional or personal agendas, quite often involving clashes of egos. She spent a lot of time conditioning her body and no time on her inner self. Linda showed Penelope the same meditation techniques she had taught Victor, as a first step towards stilling her driven mental condition, and as a means of releasing herself from the urge to be in control all the time. Periods of time spent "out of her mind" would create an oasis of calm she sorely needed for completely different reasons to Victor. Meditation, combined with visits to mosques, churches and great architectural spaces would also help to distance Penelope from the heat and immediacy of life and put her into a more reflective state; and being in the presence of calm water and in cool fresh air should become regular features of life to Penelope's Pitta constitution. Leisure time could supply all the opportunities she needed to develop this critical sense of spirit.

....and for a Kapha person. Karen's earthy Kapha nature needed no further grounding: she was already a still and calm person, reflective, caring and thoughtful. Her need to connect with that life-force outside herself could be expressed in different ways to Victor and Penelope. The avoidance of confrontation, the lack of peaks and troughs in her sensory experiences and her innate Kapha solidity required balancing with active spiritual steps. Our connection to universal energy can be found in the hills and the crashing waves as much as the churches and sacred places and for Karen a particular balance could be found in the wild places she seldom visited. Brisk walks, windy hilltops, thunder and wild seas would take her into contact with another face of spiritual awareness. Victor and Penelope's lives were already full of vigour and change and they would benefit from periods of calmness and reflection. Karen already had that therefore she would benefit from exposure to uncontrollable elemental forces. Victor's Vata type was full of air so he needed no extra shifting, changing winds, only earthy grounding experiences; Penelope's Pitta temperament was full of fiery transformational qualities so she needed no more heating up and over stimulation, only cooling calmness; Karen's Kapha nature was solid, grounded and earthy so she needed no more of those qualities, only rejuvenating vigour and welcome changeability.

Chapter 5

Making
Environmental Changes

Awareness is a word that often stimulates mixed reactions. We speak disparagingly about 'lack of awareness' when someone tramples over our feelings, and we enjoy heightened awareness when all our senses are enlivened by emotions, sensations or events. Awareness is generally recognised to be a highly desirable human attribute, something to strive for and to maintain and something that, in its sustained state, is the preserve of the few. In these pages we speak frequently of awareness as a quality that can be nurtured, something that improves our quality of existence. Improved levels of sensory awareness, like improved communicational skills, can lead to greater clarity and a better experience of life.

Awareness is seen as an aspect of consciousness and western society flatters itself into thinking that human consciousness is the supreme condition of existence. Centuries of philosophy and culture have taught us to think that these higher levels of conscious awareness are usually achieved through our thinking brain, through our mind. The problem is that the conscious mind to which we attach so much importance can process only relatively small amounts of information and deal with a only tiny percentage of the stimuli that we are exposed to. Our conscious minds have no dealings with the thousands of essential processes, reactions and responses that sustain our state of life. Subconscious processes govern all bodily functions and most of our waking activity. For most of our lives we act, speak and react without conscious effort.

We respond to our surroundings and the millions of large and small messages we receive from every facet of our environment without stopping to think simply because we couldn't deal with them all if we had to think about every one. Our central nervous systems learn the critical actions required to see, speak, eat, walk, run, throw, catch, handle tools, drive—everything we need to be able to do simply to exist. Control and co-ordination develops as we need it, through attention and practice, but we are driven for most of our lives by unconscious acts and we don't cultivate our subconscious abilities.

Together with all other creatures, humans can sense and perceive without intellectual consciousness or self-awareness. We don't need the consciousness required for intellectual debate to be able to sense things. It is a long-standing prejudice that intelligence and knowledge can only exist within the mind whereas, in fact, all living creatures sense different things relating to their environment, most of which we humans are blissfully unaware. Mammals can sense impending earthquakes and storms; trees can release substances to warn neighbours of attacks by larvae and bacteria can sense chemical differences in their surroundings; there are far too many examples of sensory perception and inherent knowledge in the plant and animal kingdoms for us to mention here. The point is that living systems are cognitive systems; living involves the process of learning and making use of acquired knowledge for all life forms

Self-awareness can be a mixed blessing. An accomplished pianist is not self-conscious when he or she plays, nor an artist when he paints or draws, nor a racing driver or tennis player or master in any discipline. Such skills are achieved by repeated practise that ultimately sidesteps conscious awareness. Very often we are our most skilful when we are least self-aware, when we lose ourselves to the instinctive acts that we have prepared for. Our subconscious intelligence and our central nervous systems allow us to 'know' without conscious effort how to exercise remarkably high levels of skill and co-ordination and how to communicate thoughts, feelings and clear verbal and non-verbal messages in an instant. In other words, excessive reverence for the western model of consciousness is a trap. We are far more than the product of conscious thought.

Many cultures encourage disrupted or diminished self-awareness. Spiritual practises encourage loss of selfhood to a greater whole. Meditation heightens consciousness by bypassing it and moving the subject to a state of "no mind." Primitive art demonstrates the level to which unconscious imagery pervaded the minds of early artists without recourse to what is now seen as conscious intelligence.

Deliberate, conscious perception accounts for only a fraction of our sensory experience most of which comes through subliminal perception. From childhood and throughout our lives we learn subliminally. Often we refer to this process as experiential learning, but much more is involved than simply participating directly in activities. Our subliminal intelligence, embedded within our subconscious, absorbs influences and information from all around us on a continual basis. We only consciously process about one millionth of the information we use daily to survive and without our subliminal intelligence we would cease to function. In one sense, consciousness allows us to choose which filters we use.

How do these two modes of intelligence affect of our quality of life and how can we use them from an Ayurvedic standpoint? We have already examined the significance of self-knowledge in relation to the tastes and the senses and this work should by now be resonating as you become more in tune with your nutritional and sensory needs. Here we'll deal with the physical environment and our response to factors that might at first appear to be out of our control. The problem is that subliminal intelligence never stops working; whilst we use conscious awareness to filter our world view, it accounts for only a fraction of our whole experience of life. Our environment is a continual source of information that affects us subliminally at the deepest level. The dark art of subliminal advertising was developed (and subsequently banned) from industry's recognition of the inherent suggestive power of subliminal imagery. Fortunately we can make conscious efforts to recognise influences, imagery, forms and artefacts for what they are and remove ourselves from potentially damaging environments and create healthier conditions to live and work in.

Whilst subliminal advertising may have been banned, the increasingly fragmentary nature of 21st Century life provides ample opportunities for impression and persuasion and the fracturing of cohesive patterns of thought. Constant saturation from sound and visual influences is a daily reality, with advertising the dominant element. By paying critical attention to the pervading influences around us and exercising choice through selective filtering, we can de-clutter our environments and increase our ability to sense the difference between harmful and beneficial influences and situations. How many homes have the TV on for more than one hour or maybe two per day? More critically, how many young children are subjected to hours of unnecessary exposure to TV, with its uncontrolled flood of sound and imagery and persuasive advertising? How many hours of gossip and hearsay do we experience in our working environment and how much negativity are we subjected to through this process? How much materialism, projection of false ideals of the body, sex, aggression and unnecessary violence are communicated through media and advertising? How much casually violent language is absorbed into daily life from sensation-based TV schedules? How much violence do we absorb through these sources and also through the vastness of the animal slaughter industry?

Our lives are saturated by coercive and carelessly destructive influences. This problem is endemic in the western world, and increasingly in the east, as global communication techniques become homogenised. Consumerism is a massive force of prodigious energy with tentacles everywhere. Most people don't know themselves well enough to know what they want and they fall for the suggestive power of the media in its many guises. Most people do not realise what suits their personality and body type, so it's small wonder that environmental stress has increased. We are rightly concerned with the state of our planet and with the crisis of global warming, but we cannot develop effective strategies for the larger problems and ignore those closer to home. We need to develop the ability to see a situation or environment for what it is and not be sucked into its false frame of reference, nor be trapped by lack of clarity about what goes on at the physical and sensory levels. We need to recognise innate qualities within different environments and equate them with our doshas in order to live more effectively. For some doshas a particular environment may be incredibly stressful and disturbing, whereas for others it might contain just the right amount of stimulation to shift moribund energies. Understanding our core needs allows us to recognise the positive and negative factors in our surroundings and act accordingly.

We witnessed a very good example of environmental confusion recently and suffered the consequences, so it's worth describing this typical situation in some detail, because you will all have had similar experiences; the experience allowed us to observe ourselves in what became a surprisingly uncomfortable situation.

A new bookshop opened close to where Linda lives and works. It is part of a chain, had a large stock of books, CD's and other media and, most importantly, it had a café serving good coffee. One of life's great pleasures is to browse through books, buy something interesting and then sit and read it over coffee and carrot cake, or a sandwich. Sometimes you can break through a minor blockage or clear your head simply by leaving the office and surrounding yourself with thousands of pages of other people's thoughts and words. That's what we planned, and we took ourselves down there with a notebook and pen intending to do some work at the same time.

The place was quite crowded, but we found a spare table, got our food and drink and sat down to work. We do this often in a different bookshop and anticipated a good time here in the new venue. Very quickly we realised that this was not as good a location as we had hoped. The first thing we noticed was the rapid turnaround of customers. They were consuming their food and drinks and leaving quickly. This is what they were supposed to do. What at face value had seemed to be a well-designed, attractive space had, it seemed, actually been designed to accommodate people in only relative comfort. The colour scheme, furniture and flooring all conspired to move them on. A seemingly stylish and homely meeting place had all the factors that make a ten-minute stay seem just about enough.

The walls were deep burgundy contrasted with olive green. This is an active combination of colours, more subtle that the glaring contrasts of some other retail outlets and fast food chains, but just as effective in creating a vaguely uncomfortable backdrop to the rest of the layout. Red is a colour that heats up a room and even in this more restrained variation it was potent. Olive green, though relatively muted is a powerful complimentary to the red, and the two colours, in the large amounts within this space, fought for dominance. That is what complimentary colours do. The flooring was hard: functional, modern but spartan. The furniture was wooden, dark mahogany in colour, but sparsely styled, utilitarian rather than rustic, which was the implied theme, and of mean proportions. Wooden furniture promises natural qualities, comfort and a certain unity but these chairs and tables didn't work. The chairs didn't have flowing shapes or ergonomics and were uncomfortable.

The space was open plan and the serving counter was of glass and stainless steel. At a glance the combined impression was sophisticated and attractive. However, sound levels were high and harsh, crockery rattled and clattered behind the counter and the air conditioning was blowing too fiercely. Everywhere we looked there were hard edges and angles and what had appeared to be a comfortable, well-planned space turned out to be quite the opposite. We were influenced by the impression of professionalism and an implied sense of relaxation but the place failed to live up to its promise.

In these circumstances it would have been easy to blame the bank holiday crowds and put our struggle to work down to deficiencies on our part, but the fact was that we had chosen the wrong place to do what we wanted to do. Appearances had deceived us and, having realised that, we were free to make a new choice.

Our senses provided the tools that led to this realisation and they will do the same for you too. When entering into any situation or environment run through a checklist, led by the senses of **sight, touch, sound and spirit**. Make the conscious effort to recognise what is going on around you. Ask yourself:

- How does it look? Describe your surroundings to yourself; describe the floors, furniture, walls, displays and purpose of the space you are in. Describe the colours, shapes and patterns you see.

- How does it feel? Use your whole body, use your hands and use your eyes to describe the shapes, textures and range of surfaces around you. Are there regular or irregular spaces between the objects in front of you and how do they relate to human scale?

- How does it sound? Close your eyes and describe the quality of sound. Is there silence? Are there voices and if so are they a soft murmur, loud and happy, angry and argumentative, aggressive, commanding? Can you hear machinery of any kind, is it obtrusive and can you hear other unwelcome noises?

- How does it feel? Be still and allow yourself to recognise what the situation is creating inside you. How do you feel about your immediate surroundings—comfortable or uncomfortable, neutral or otherwise? Are you relaxed or stimulated, and if stimulated is this a positive or a negative sensation? Do you feel any particular energy from the place and the people in it?

These questions are the basis for an appraisal of any environment you move into. We will now look in more detail at the factors that affect our three case studies, and a table that provides basic guidance notes for working with your respective living, working and leisure environments can be found in Appendix E.

Let's return to our starting point and examine the physical and sensory factors within the immediate working and home environments of Victor, Penelope and Karen.

Working environment

Victor

Victor's working space was visually stimulating. He worked in the Graphic Design industry, in the company of many other designers, using a variety of technologies. Ongoing photographic and design processes surrounded him and, not only did he work on his Apple Mac and create great visual material, he was also completely immersed in imagery from the output of his colleagues. His Vata vision was saturated with colours, shapes and light emanating from computer screens and hard copies of their work. The studio was clean and quite new with numerous drawing tables, workstations, notice boards, displays and PR material and it was a hot house of creativity driven by deadlines and the continual expansion of workloads. Victor never stopped to give his eyes a break. He was either on line, pushing software to its limits and making continual demands on his visual faculties, or guiding colleagues in their own design work. He looked at everything that came his way filling his hard drive with source material and half finished ideas for projects. His workspace was full of postcards and clippings that he'd collected and he existed in a kaleidoscopic environment.

In tactile terms Victor experienced a more limited range of sensations. The studio was rich in colour, light and shape but less so in texture. There was a "virtual" feel to the workspace and in fact more pictures of texture than actual texture. Besides the computers, lighting and cameras, aluminium and glass were the dominant materials, very chic, very sleek and very expensive, but lacking natural warmth and real world texture. In fact most surfaces were eerily smooth, apart from the occasional jumble of papers or proofs on desks. Even the office walls and partitions were glass. There was a lot of style and panache, but no plants, no roughness, no earthy qualities anywhere.

Sound levels were intense. There was constant discussion and conversation, banter and joking when things were going well and curses and rage when things went wrong. No particular sound was excessive but the layers of interacting communication were very distracting; the hyped up atmosphere, fostered by management and key staff, kept designers on their toes, not that they needed encouraging. Phone calls were constant and conversations took place over the full width of the studio as clients' requests were checked with other contributors. Added to this was a background noise from the FM radio station and the sound of printers whirring and clattering. The stimulation in this environment was beginning to be too much for Victor's unbalanced Vata state.

Victor felt distracted before he even walked into work. Driving through heavy traffic is something that many people have to do, and we can see the effects of these levels of stress all too easily. Once in place, Victor slipped immediately into a reactive mode of activity. He responded to every email, every design problem, every question from his boss or his colleagues and every phone call. His creative brain, his vision and his skilled hands were never at rest and, even when active within the design process, he responded to stimuli or queries outside his immediate frame of reference.

What should Victor do?

Victor needed to create stillness within the shifting visual, auditory and tactile bedlam of his workplace. His Vata mind needed respite from all the stimulation, and he needed a means of anchoring himself in the moment that would allow clarity of thought and some inner peace. He couldn't take control of the whole environment, but he could manage his own immediate space and he could take some important steps towards managing input from external sources. There was also quite a degree of autonomy in terms of dress code, informal relationships between staff and management and personal working space, so Victor had some scope for change.

Victor was a real technophile and the sound issues presented him with a perfect excuse to use his iPod. Rather than play the dance music he usually turned to, he could download chants, mantras, orchestral music, a classical repertoire, choral sounds and a wealth of material that would calm his Vata mind. This would put an effective soundtrack between him and the bustle of the office without cutting him off completely. He might even try changing the station on the office radio.

He could reduce the visual stimuli around his immediate working area and introduce a limited number of new images showing peaceful scenes. He could set aside a special place on his desk that was uncluttered and had the sole function of representing stillness to him; that spot needed rocks, wood, ceramics or a live plant, items that were not "virtual" and would become his grounding point. He needed to separate the various aspects of his work so that emails were only responded to at certain intervals, allowing him more time to concentrate on one thing at a time.

He and everyone else in the office needed some exposure to real natural texture, so he could approach his boss with a view to bringing in some live plants and gravel bed displays for them. Natural wood, unvarnished, even bleached like driftwood, grasses and real earthy qualities were needed. Even if they had to rely on photographs of these things, that would be an improvement. The images needed to be large enough to have presence and to establish the feeling of an oasis within the heated creative sphere they all worked in. Victor's desk images would be of similar subject matter.

Since he was Mr Techno personified, Victor could also get a suitable screensaver that would continue to remind him of the need for some regulation and tranquillity in his daily life.

Penelope

Penelope's working spaces were utilitarian, spiced by the clamour provided by 2000 children as they changed classes six times a day. The school had never been refurbished and showed signs of wear and tear. Fluorescent lights, discontinuity of colour schemes, cluttered desks in staff rooms, a hotchpotch of furniture and overflowing notice boards defined the visual style. Working surfaces and seating arrangements were ad hoc, with no consistency of size or type; computers were crammed onto desks and filing cabinets fitted uncomfortably into any available space. Some attempts had been made to introduce artwork created by students but there weren't the resources to frame things properly, so displays soon became tatty. A large meeting room was the only space which had any sense of visual order and that was largely because it wasn't required to store or display information. Variety can be stimulating, but what Penelope and the other staff experienced was visual anarchy; there were no unifying themes throughout the school.

The tactile sensations provided by the mass of paper-based information, by the piles of students' work assembled for marking, by the irregularity of desks, cupboards and cabinets and by the utilitarian corridors were confusing and unfriendly. In ergonomic terms, the only spaces in the school that worked were the craft workshops and domestic science areas, which were fitted out to make safe and effective use of space and equipment; and the frequently used computer suite, which had been purpose designed. The rest of the physical environment was dominated by the texture of wood veneer or plastic surfaces, with no natural textures; the overriding sensation was of irregularity and discomfort.

Sound levels were relatively high between lessons and acceptably low during lessons. This range is not surprising, and corridor management, with all the potential for conflict entailed by the movement of large numbers of young people was part of Penelope's role in the school day. Within each classroom annoying scrapes and creaks created by chairs being moved were the source of tension for all staff as they pursued the dual goals of education and classroom management. Overall sound levels were not high in an industrial sense, but the nature and source of each sound, arising as they did from restlessness on the part of the pupils, added to the tension that exists in many teaching situations. Sound, other than during discussions in classes and staff meetings, usually represented potential conflict and as such it created anxiety. When silence occurred it was very welcome.

Even before interacting with her working spaces Penelope felt overheated and tense. The quiet periods when she could simply get on with teaching or administration were offset by her general discomfort created by all the nutritional and other factors in her life, and especially by the tension that existed in her management role, dealing as she did with difficult issues and difficult staff. Her lack of patience with staff who resisted new developments in curriculum delivery, together with the re-structuring currently underway in the school, manifested itself in many ways. Confrontation and arguments with staff were matched by the incessant pace of her life. There was no emotional or physical stability in her working environment. As her stress levels crept up they were like a worm inside her and each problem, each aspect of her surroundings aggravated her to a disproportionate degree making her Pitta fire flare up. Then she would drink more coffee and fuel the fire, and meetings would become confrontations.

What should Penelope do?

She couldn't rebuild the school or buy new equipment and she was doing everything possible, as an effective manager of young people around the buildings, to keep noise levels within acceptable limits. However she could begin to transform her own immediate working space. She could use her authority to set up better display systems and she could organise a rota that maintained only the necessary minimum amount of information around the school and staff rooms. Alignment of visual displays so that, for instance, the tops of all pages displayed were at a constant level would help remove the impression of chaos. Colour coding would also unify this visual material.

She could survey the existing furniture and relocate similar types to create "family groups" for specific areas. She could organise support staff to place plants and flowers in key spaces around the school. She could ask Art Department staff to organise tactile wall hangings, bringing new creative sources of stimulation, and they might also be colour coordinated to suit their surroundings.

Sound levels were not as excessive as some environments, and Penelope handled the movements along corridors efficiently. The shuffles and scrapes of classroom life fell within the teacher's domain, but she could support them by making unwelcome classroom noise more of an issue during assemblies. Loose and squeaking hinges, and the noise caused by wear and tear, could be dealt with by caretaking staff and Penelope could choose to prioritise this work. The dining room was noisy with occasional eruptions of mayhem and Penelope could consider introducing a unifying low volume sound track to level out the atmosphere. Meditation CD's, classical music and chants have a strong soothing effect on everyone. This music could even be used in staff rooms as low background sound.

She had plenty to work on with her new Ayurvedic approach to self-care, much of which we have examined already. However Penelope needed to take specific measures to deal with her feelings within her professional environment.

- Taking five minutes to use the three-part breathing technique at critical moments (see Appendix F) would immediately reduce her stress levels.

- Walking slowly in the school grounds, breathing fresh air and feeling natural light on her skin would relieve tension and stimulate skin tone.

- Buying sweet smelling flowers for her desk would soothe her Pitta heat.

- Using aromatherapy oils would ground and calm her Pitta energy.

Karen

Karen's working environment was visually restrained. It was ordered, well laid out and ergonomically efficient. Colours were neutral, with warm greys, lighter tints and some lavender highlights. Everyone worked at a desk, with a flat screen computer, in- and out-trays, a desk organiser, calendar and company notepads. Modern filing cabinets with discreet sliding doors punctuated the space around desks in a regulated fashion. Venetian blinds screened excess light levels, so that computer screens were more visible and the overhead lighting was of high quality. There were spotlights over a meeting area, which added a tasteful note of contrast. Furniture, desks, partitions and notice boards were of one style with no incongruities, and the only hint of visual anarchy came from what people chose to wear or pin to their desk-side pin boards. Some of the staff had brought photographs and toys or mascots to their workstations, and Karen had a calendar with 'nice country views'. The overall effect in the office was calming, a quality that would have been good for Penelope. Ironically, Penelope's working conditions, or indeed Victor's would have been good for Karen.

The tactile experience within this homogenous environment was almost as tasteful as its visual appearance. Carpeted floors, adjustable swivel chairs and properly functioning workspaces meant that each employee was comfortable. There were no extremes of shape or angle to disturb their touch sensors or their eyes. Paperwork was either kept in trays awaiting processing or filed away out of sight. Desks were regularly spaced with dividers of consistent heights, combined with a repeating textural motif of plastic edged veneers; there were hessian seat covers, plastic screens and computer casings. which were the only tactile sensation besides the clothes that people wore. One large plant in a corner of the office provided the only hint of disarray. There were no other natural references other than picture calendars.

Sound levels were low. Conversation was not forbidden, but the work required concentration and people only spoke to each other casually between longer periods of quietness. Telephones were not busy, since this was not a sales office, and neither music nor radios were allowed. Traffic noise was too distant to be a nuisance and the only consistent noise was the hum of computers. A meeting room provided a discreet space for discussion between managers and staff. In most ways this was a good working environment.

Karen was stuck in a rut and she knew it. Her working environment was comfortable and she had been able to avoid some of the challenges that came with her role. She was unhappy at the prospect of changes she would have to implement but had been able to avoid taking action up to now. She was a keen advocate of the concept of leaving things until tomorrow and the quietness and order of the office provided a good hiding place. She was able to maintain a monotonous level of pro-activity through the technicalities of her work that left the physical and emotional status quo of the whole office environment untouched. She kept her head down; hoped things would go away; and merged into the blandness of her surroundings. There was very little excitement through her senses of sight, touch and sound and she actually couldn't be bothered to make the effort to change things.

What should Karen do?

Karen's working environment would, in many ways, be the envy of many. Calmness and order were tangible through the physical details of the office and the nature of the work she undertook. Things were always controlled. The equipment, furniture and décor were all of good quality, in good condition and caused no physical stress to anyone. Nothing distracted her from her computer screen, or the files and paperwork that she took from their nicely appointed spaces, as she needed them. The scene resembled a film set for the office version of the Stepford Wives, with restraint and evenness the overriding characteristic. To someone in Karen's unbalanced Kapha condition, such anonymous comfort (and apparent security) was a refuge she didn't need.

Karen needed to shift and raise her energy levels. She needed stimulation. Within the office, although there were limitations imposed by the nature of the work, she could still bring about some useful changes to her immediate visual experience. Karen needed contrasts; she needed bold tones and accents of stronger colours that would spice things up. She could also extend these effects to other parts of the office too, and she could do this by introducing powerful architectural images, bold carnival scenes and crisp images of food, flowers and street scenes. These images could come from calendars and posters but could involve the staff who, although reluctant to move to new work roles, would benefit from more direct involvement with Karen at any level. She could get them to contribute to the visual and tactile themes she would introduce.

Sound and touch: Linda suggested bringing some Japanese elements into her working space, with stones and fine gravel to create crunchy textures and sounds that would be perfect for stimulating Karen's senses. Bonsai trees or a miniature garden would be great. Tactile experiences from urban locations with their particular textures ranging from chrome to the coarsest building materials were excellent for energising her Kapha temperament. Walking through city streets, feeling her own pace and the bustle of other people brushing by would be powerful experiences for her. She needed to find pavement cafes and similarly lively settings where she could feel new, urban sensations. Lunchtimes could be spent on lively forays away from the office even if only twenty minutes were available.

Home environment

Any examination of our environment should involve the holistic consideration that we are all part of the spaces we inhabit. We bring our inner condition and ourselves to our observation of everything around us. The factors that affect our sense of wellbeing interact and we cannot be divorced from our inner feelings when we respond to our surroundings. Nutrition helps us to recreate each cell of our bodies and in the instant of seeing and feeling, our nutrition and its rightness for our dosha affect our perception. Our responses are affected by the inner levels of balance and harmony; if we are highly charged emotionally our responses will be different from when we are calm and capable of reflection. So, nutrition and meditation form the cornerstone to our inner state of mind, regardless of our dosha. No matter what changes we make to our outer environment they are wasted if we fail to make maintain our inner space. Nutrition and meditation are the building blocks for everything else we do.

We have examined in detail the working environments of our three case studies; what you have learned here is transferable to any other place you find yourself. Solving the complexity and conflicts found at work makes home life much easier to deal with. Home is where the most effective changes can be made without constraint. What follows is a description of the most beneficial sounds, colours and shapes for each dosha. They apply to Victor, Penelope and Karen and they apply to you. When you have read through the descriptions you don't need to rush around redecorating or do anything drastic. Changes can be incremental and you can use accessories and accents of colour and texture to introduce the new elements that you'll now begin to learn about.

Sound type and quality can be dealt with immediately. In Chapter 4 we looked at the sense of hearing and the same considerations apply in this broader environmental context. Of concern is the type and quality of sound within the home and work place. Making changes at home and, where possible, at work creates powerful support systems for your dosha. Sound type, quality and volume have profound effects on our wellbeing. We should never put up with damaging sound and we should always strive to improve our auditory input. Here are some general principles for the three doshas:

Vata: sounds should be warm, consistent, soothing and softer in tone and should help to calm the mind. All sound, music and mantras should not be too loud and should not continue for long periods as it depletes Vata energy.

Pitta: sounds should be cool, soothing, calming and not demanding. Mantras, chants and spiritual music are great for Pitta.

Kapha: sounds of strong vocal singing and chanting with warm, stimulating and activating tones are all great for Kapha.

Classical music harms nobody and Vata and Pitta types especially benefit from listening to it and also to incantatory music, chants, choral sounds, drones and harmonies and spiritual music. These are calming sounds for Vata and Pitta doshas, and thus not ideal for Kapha all of the time. Kapha types need livelier music of any kind to invigorate them. At home none of this is a problem, because each type can play the best music for them, but work or family life with different doshas around always requires compromise. With this in mind let us re-state that variety is better for everyone than too much of the wrong stuff. Remember that no music is banned; we can enjoy whatever form of music we like in a balanced way.

Colours

Here are some pointers for all doshas to work with to promote harmony in the home, based on the science of colour therapy. Like sound, colour has a profound effect on our emotions and our health. Remember the experience we described in the bookshop café. The subliminal signals from colour schemes are incredibly persuasive, so learning some of the underlying principles will be of enormous benefit to you and all around you.

Before we look at each dosha here are some general ideas:

- Use coloured bulbs or cover lamps with the relevant coloured cloth to create change.

- Remove all fluorescent lights as these have bad effects on all doshas.

- Use daylight bulbs and full spectrum lighting in the winter to relieve all doshas of winter blues.

- Choose as many natural colours as possible within your home environment.

- Add natural colours through flowers, plants and crystals for work environments where possible.

- Use a background of light but neutral shades to work alongside the specific dosha colours. For suitable colours for each dosha, see below.

Vata: the best colours are golds, yellows, emerald green, sky blue, reds, oranges and pink. Stick with the warmer tones keeping cooler ones to a minimum.

Avoid bright and flashy purples, reds, or too much by way of deep and dark colours.

Pitta: the best colours are whites, all greens, blues, silvers and soft shades and pastels. Pitta people love contrasts and will use opposites to create drama and although this is good in a balanced Pitta, it will not help when Pitta is aggravated.

Avoid reds, oranges, golds and yellows.

Kapha: the best colours are strong reds, oranges, yellows and golds with some contrasts. These stimulate Kapha and create movement; be careful not to overdo this and create chaos that might lead to a feeling of being overwhelmed.

Avoid whites, pinks and pale colours, all of which encourage lethargy in an already stable dosha type.

Here are some general guidelines for using Ayurvedic colour theory

Grey: creates neutrality helps to reduce emotional charge—but for a low energy person it can create depression.

Brown: helps to stabilise as it is an earth colour and works well with a contrasting enlivening colour in the same way that green grass and flowers work with brown in nature.

Red: increases warmth, power and energy, but can promote hostility, anger and aggravation.

Yellow: stimulates intelligence, but can be too much for an already over-stimulated or agitated mind.

Green: promotes harmony, calms the mind and nerves, but will increase Kapha qualities if used in excess. Note: this is why it is used in hospitals, but it can also be detrimental inducing boredom. This colour requires accessorising.

Blue: helps create a sense of solitude and meditation, but can sometimes feel cold and unfriendly.

Purple: has the effect of creating a cold sense of distance and authority. With certain textures, silk for example, it creates sensual but 'wicked' undertones. Purple can encourage inner angst and suppress emotions.

Gold: harmonises the mind and strengthens energy.

White: provides nurturing pure properties, but can add to cool and lethargic states.

Black: can be overbearing and creates a sense of heaviness or even menace in large amounts, but can add impact as an accessory. This colour is associated with death.

Colour and texture have obvious qualities. What may be less obvious is how we perceive the shapes and forms of our surroundings. Regardless of the function of objects in our environment we are affected by their formal or geometric properties. We respond directly to the hardness or softness, the roundness or squareness, the curved and the angular things in our homes, work and in public places. Here are some guidelines on shapes that will help you implement changes in re-arranging your home.

Shapes and forms that suit each Dosha type

Shapes have the two-dimensional properties of height and width and differ from form, which has the additional property of depth. Our initial recognition of form, however, is through shape and the outline of an object or a location is powerfully suggestive. Interior walls and ceilings, known to architects as planes, exert powerful influences on our sensibilities. They interact to create active or passive elements, forming barriers that limit our movement but creating opportunities for enclosure and for circulation between separate elements. Floors support us, walls enclose us and ceilings, usually out of touch, provide shelter and define the limits of a structure. Each of these three kinds of planes can be coloured and textured to modify their influence. In combination, these three planes form the compositions that we live in, and as we move from one environment to another our perceptions alter according to the qualities and proportions of wall, floors and ceilings. When we are outside, in nature or in the city, we still respond to the ground plane, the 'ceiling' plane of the sky and the vertical and diagonal planes of landscape or architecture. We are actually surrounded by a shifting series of compositions within which we act out our lives.

Diagonal arrangements and compositions, whether they are two or three-dimensional stimulate a sense of movement and dynamism. Horizontal and vertical combinations stimulate a sense of order. If we were to place these contrasting themes in an architectural context, classical stability comes in the form of Greek temples; restless energy and a sense of movement comes in the form of many of the great structures in concrete, or post-modern extremes of styling. On the High Street, classical imagery implies quality and reliability. In contrast, advertising imagery, displays and the prevalence of graphics and media stimulate movement, enquiry and action on the part of us consumers.

It is surprising how deeply our appreciation of the cultural inheritance of classical proportions and principles is felt. We have already discussed the Golden Section and the Fibonacci Series, ratios that exist throughout the natural world, and their continuing effect on how we respond to our environment. These effects are felt through an intuitive understanding of structures. Lintels and upright arrangements that we see in any doorway or window form the basis for our grassroots understanding of stabilising forces. We are completely familiar with the logic of this balance of elements and from childhood we carry this sense of why things stand upright from our explorations with building blocks and from the walls, pillars and posts around us. The sense of stability is reinforced throughout our lives whenever an element such as a vertical column, window feature or doorway is repeated, or whenever we create a pattern by placing pictures on a wall.

Any diagonal line, shape of structure brings a tension to that inbuilt logic. Diagonal lines are dynamic and visually active. When architects and civil engineers could shake off the restraints imposed by traditional building materials and make full use of concrete building technology in the early 20th Century, new structures could then be created that brought curved planes into play in ways that were previously impossible. Le Corbusier, the great Modernist architect and designer, used the full potential of concrete to create structures that not only maintained classical proportions, but also which explored the potential of vast curved planes. Nervi, the great Italian architect, created huge domes that utilised the strength and lightness of concrete and which also tease our sense of the possible. On the grand scale that architects have worked at it is inspiring to feel the effect of planes, forms and shapes in space, but the same potential exists in the smallest location. Within any environment there are many possible variations of composition, of arrangement and the layout of elements. We grow by knowing what effects they have on us. In landscapes, horizontal ground planes and sky planes dominate. We compare angles of steepness with our horizon. When we experience sustained diagonal planes from close up, as when climbing a steep mountainside, they have a pronounced effect that makes surrounding space all the more keenly felt.

We identify and characterise form by recognising shape. Shape refers to lines and contours that limit a figure, or form. The qualities of shapes around us create feeling and reactions that make us comfortable or uncomfortable. We should become aware of the shape, size, colour and texture of our surroundings, actual spaces we are in and the objects within them. We should be aware of the position and orientation of these objects. We respond instinctively to objects within our visual field in terms of their primary geometric qualities, so that circular, triangular and square shapes and forms are the bedrock of our experience; they are defined by the spaces that surround them. Recognising these basic geometric boundaries helps us to regulate our domestic environments. We can add elements to create changes, or we can subtract them.

Vata: should introduce rounded shapes, square balanced shapes, and soft textures and forms into their environment to calm the Vata system. These changes will help release the emotions of fear and anxiety and encourage a feeling of peace and harmony in life and your home.

Pitta: can choose work with all shapes and forms but try to avoid sharp hard angles. Following this rule you will find that your heated aggravation decreases, resentment and impatience subside, bringing about calm, compassion and forgiveness.

Kapha: try to avoid circular, round or square shapes and forms, try using angular, pyramid shapes for a sense of movement. You will see a relaxing of greedy emotion, obsessive feelings of attachment and develop more clarity and energy.

Everyone should consider the qualities of the colours and shapes around them and adapt their home environment to help balance their dosha. When you take the environment and the senses into consideration you can bring about positive change to your dosha imbalances. Working with these colour themes, with shape and the senses will enhance the transformation already taking place as a result of increased awareness combined with nutritional and sensory changes. Spending leisure time planning the changes will increase balance in all doshas.

Chapter 6

Sleep and Relaxation

What is sleep?

In Ayurveda sleep is believed to connect us to our ancestral roots, when we strengthen the crucial sense of who we are and where we come from. We connect to the greater environment and to a pulse of energy common to all living creatures following the great sequence of circadian and seasonal rhythms. In sleep we leave conscious activity behind.

People usually think of sleep as a time when all activity stops, a period when we shut down completely to allow our bodies to recuperate. It's true that during sleep our metabolism changes and our bodies relax, but our brains actually shift to another mode of activity. In sleep the brain releases hormones that stimulate cellular activity throughout the body and our brain waves actually indicate more activity than during waking hours, burning large quantities of sugar and oxygen. We go through essential phases of sleep, each showing different kinds of brain waves and we dream even if we don't always remember what occurred in the dreams. All of this is vital to physical and emotional health. One of the critical phases, REM (Rapid Eye Movement) sleep, which occurs in all species, appears to be crucial to developing infants and adults alike, since during this phase brain cells are renewed.

We need sleep to function properly and we cannot sleep without having been awake! Our body's cycles of waking and sleeping are as natural as night and day and we have biological clocks that tick away our daily allocation of wakefulness. William Dement, arguably the world's leading researcher on the subject of sleep, describes all wakefulness as sleep deprivation. He believes that our bodies monitor our hours of wakefulness that need repaying with corresponding levels of sleep at an approximate ration of 1:2. On this basis we need about 8 hours sleep every night.

We are no different from our ancestors in the need for sleep, despite 24-hour access to light, food and comfort. Like our ancestors, we are natural creatures in a natural world that is subject to daily and seasonal rhythms. Mother Earth provides us with everything we need and natural cycles create life, crop growth, weather and the larger environment that we inhabit. We are integral to all life around us, but technology has skewed our sense of what is natural. We sleep less than all previous generations, on average one and a half hours less per night than people a century ago. We live in a faster paced, and in many ways, more demanding society than all previous ones, without the benefit of enough sleep for our natural biological needs. Artificial light, intrusive media and television, continual access to information and fragmented work patterns all disrupt our body's natural rhythms. Vast numbers of people under-perform and live miserable lives simply because they ignore or fail to understand their body's needs and they often live with severe sleep deprivation. Increases in working hours and gradual changes to life in general are robbing us of the sleep we need. Not only do we work longer hours, we follow active leisure and family pursuits that eat away at the time available for proper amounts of sleep. External influences tempt us into believing that action is better than contemplation, that movement is better than stillness. These influences are many and varied: shops, bars and clubs open late, the boundaries of holiday periods are crossed and when we are at home 24-hour stimulation is readily available to gnaw away at the time available one of the most essential processes for the health of our bodies.

There is a cultural aspect to making do with less sleep and we are encouraged to marvel at world leaders or giants of industry who work one hundred hours a week. Western culture disrespects sleep and yet sleep deprivation is a killer. We have all experienced periods of daytime drowsiness and the effect it has on our work. Efficiency and the ability to perform simple, let alone complex tasks requiring physical and mental co-ordination are severely affected by lack of sleep, and fatigue and drowsiness can have dramatic effects, causing car crashes and other catastrophic events. Fatigue can even lead to heart disease and the erosion of essential bodily functions.

Sleep disorders worldwide cost billions of pounds and dollars per year and are largely created by ignorance of natural rhythms and cycles. As recently as 100 years ago people were exposed to less light and less stimulation than we are nowadays. Midnight was the middle of the night because people went to bed earlier, woke earlier and more slowly, and they adhered to more natural daily patterns of activity. That is no longer the case and post-industrial societies around the world follow the western way in extending days that obliterate the sequences of light and dark that are programmed into our genetic code.

Excessive and extended levels of light and stimulation combine to undermine our body clocks, which maintain alertness and which are regulated by the circadian rhythms of night and day. We are highly responsive to light and if we expose ourselves to even relatively low levels of light later in our day, we effectively delay our biological clocks and remain alert longer than we should. This is where sleeping problems originate for most people. We fall out of synchronization with the natural cycles and develop sleep debt that cannot easily be overcome.

Although this may seem obvious now, it was not until fairly recently that scientific links between daytime sleepiness and performance were identified. There is a very clear correlation between the highest level of alertness, and the quality and type of sleep, and also between poor performance, drowsiness and low quality sleep. We are programmed to be awake in the day and asleep in the night. Our bodies automatically register the hours of wakefulness and require appropriate levels of sleep to compensate at the approximate ratio of two hours of waking time to one hour of sleep, hence the needed eight hours of sleep described earlier. We have a fascinating system of regulatory mechanisms to ensure that we feel tired enough to fall asleep after being awake for the allotted number of (daylight) hours, and that we respond internally to natural daily fluctuations in tiredness with corresponding waves of wakefulness that allow us to complete our waking day even when we have the afternoon dip in energy common to most humans. When fatigued we can rise to the occasion to complete specific tasks and achieve temporary victory over drowsiness but we can never escape the need to get enough sleep. When we fail to meet that requirement, fatigue continues to slow down our wits and reflexes, lowers our performance level,and affects our thinking and our emotional state. The longer we are awake the quicker we fall asleep to the point that alertness evaporates completely with extreme sleep deprivation.

The hours of sleep debt builds up over several days during the week and it is impossible to repay these hours with just a weekend's lie-in. The debt remains and our bodies suffer as a consequence. Researchers believe that short naps are not enough; we need to repay the sleep debt in sufficiently large increments. One good night's sleep does not replace the kind of sustained loss of sleep created by over-long workdays combined with high levels of partying! The extent to which sleep debt accrues over weeks and months is not clear, although there are some indications that over a two-week period we seem to absorb some level of drowsiness. However, sustained fatigue of this kind continues to harm our physical and emotional health, creating moods, illness and potentially long term damage. Temporary stimulation from coffee, alcohol and TV (or other bright light) doesn't actually help and the fact remains that we need more sleep than we get. Tests reinforce the predictable revelation that our health and mood improves with regular levels of good quality sleep. We can work off sleep debt, regain balance and function effectively with an average of eight hours sleep per night.

We actually need some sleep debt to be able to fall asleep and sleep debt's positive aspect accumulates during waking hours, creating the necessary level of tiredness that brings sleep. The problem we encounter is that the unaddressed sleep debt carries over from one night to another becoming a burden that some cope with better than others, but it always remains until we redress the balance with sleep. Our internal alertness mechanism may temporarily override feelings of tiredness, but the underlying fatigue remains. Whenever we feel drowsy, whenever we yawn or whenever we lose track of our thinking, we are likely to be in sleep debt sufficient to create dangerous situations when driving or doing repetitive, potentially hazardous tasks.

Our internal clock regulates our lives, controlling eating, sleeping and waking, our capacity to work, to think and to respond emotionally to our surroundings. Being diurnal creatures we are regulated by the twenty four-hour circadian rhythm of night and day. Circadian rhythms are involved in almost every bodily function. They exist at the level of basic cellular processes and at the level of whole body activities and patterns. Tests indicate that within this twenty four-hour period, primates, including man, compress their daily sleep into eight hours and wakefulness into sixteen hours. Our body clocks, in combination with accumulating sleep debt, sustain this rhythm. Other species have different responses to circadian rhythms and have different periods of sleep and wakefulness.

Sleep scientists have discovered relatively recently that our biological clock, which is remarkably accurate, is actually a light monitor that makes us alert during daylight hours. It stimulates wakefulness and it does so at critical times during a twenty four-hour period. Research has shown that although sunlight, the strongest light source we receive, is the prime regulator, we can also be affected over time by lower levels of light, and even by the low light of single light bulbs. Light resets our body clock every day, and we feel its effects even through our skin. We don't have to see it to be affected by it, since changes felt by our skin transmit the critical messages to our brain that maintain the ticking of our clock. This clock wakes us, even at weekends when we could stay in bed;it creates jet lag when our body clocks are out of sync with changed surroundings and different time-zones; it then stimulates us to remain awake despite the effects of jet lag, and to become alert in the brightness of artificial light (when at home we would be asleep), and despite sleep debt. It is a survival mechanism that maintains alertness and the capacity to function within the framework of our "normal" day.

A parallel process within our brains known as sleep homeostasis regulates sleep. When we get less sleep than we need, this homeostatic process drives us to fall asleep. When we achieve extra sleep the same process decreases our tendency to fall asleep. It seems that this process maintains an accurate record of how much sleep we have and also maintains a constant internal environment that includes body temperature and calorie intake.

The biological clock opposes this sleep tendency, maintaining alertness, but it is not continuous. The clock has two waves of activity; one which wakes us in the morning, and the other which stimulates us in the late afternoon. The later period appears to be the strongest, because as sleep debt accumulates we need greater stimulation to remain awake. In Dement's opinion early afternoon tiredness is not due to the effects of lunch, but to a biological rhythm. We are programmed by nature to wake and then re-awaken at fairly precise intervals during our day. Typical timings would be a prime period of wakefulness at nine o'clock, followed by a later and initially stronger period, when we gain our second wind, which gains strength from around six to nine o'clock in the evening. After that, sleep debt overcomes the wakening effect of our biological clock and we become tired enough to sleep. From an Ayurvedic viewpoint incorrect nutrition can certainly induce lethargy and an inability to function correctly and the Ayurvedic day has distinct phases in which one dosha predominates, creating variations in wakefulness and lethargy. These phases are discussed in Chapter 8.

In a world dominated by artificial light, we seem to run close to a twenty five-hour day, since the electric light we are exposed to resets our biological clock. We tend to stay up later, gradually accumulating sleep debt and create the Monday morning feeling of being too tired to get up even though we have had two lie-ins over the weekend. It's a fact that we receive less sleep than our great-grandparents, who had less exposure to artificial light. The first light bulb wasn't invented until 1879, but by the early nineteen hundreds bright light was available to all. Since then daytime is no longer confined to the sunlight hours and our patterns of sleep and wakefulness have shifted, but not our inner circadian rhythms. Without electric light and even now when we go off into nature, bedtime is governed by the time of sunset. In typical urban environments however, the day has shifted for millions in the post-industrialized world, and longer working days eat into the hours of darkness, extended by relaxation periods sustained in artificial light, TV schedules and travel itineraries all combining to shift bedtime to much later than in the past. For thousands of years we would have slept from perhaps eight at night until the early hours of dawn (eight hours); we would have awoken slowly and have had a long daylight-governed day. Now we go to bed late, and shock ourselves awake with alarm clocks before rushing out to work.

Although technology allows us to create our own virtual worlds, bathed in light and surrounded by stimulation, we are natural creatures with a genetic inheritance governed by circadian rhythms and by natural forces. We cannot escape this legacy. In Ayurveda sleep is a critical component of the daily pattern of life. It is part of a great planetary cycle in which we leave our conscious state and allow our larger unconscious intelligence to continue operating unhindered. In sleep we work through issues that we haven't faced or been able to deal with during the day and dreams and awakenings give us the opportunity to resolve problems that we have failed to notice or deal with during the conscious element of our day. The internal spiritual side of sleep enables emotions to be balanced and is essential to our emotional health.

The daily cycle of light and darkness has within it key periods when sleep is better achieved, and when other processes including work and also relaxation are best suited to each dosha. We sleep to recover from the efforts of the day and to allow our bodies to rebuild. This process reconnects us to our unconscious inner selves and with the collective energy that lies outside our individual selves and which forms part of a much larger whole. Sleep can be a blessed relief, something that embraces us and removes tiredness, anxiety and stress. For this to occur we should be willing to prepare for it in just the same way we prepare for any of the other critical processes in our lives.

Timing and preparation are as essential to sleep as they are to eating or any other activity, and yet they are usually overlooked. We know that to get the best out of our food we need to concentrate on how we prepare it, cook and eat it and we know that if we eat when we're in an emotionally disturbed condition we will receive less nourishment from our food. This is a critical point. No matter how good the quality of the food, or the cooking, it won't do its job properly if we are disturbed or upset.

So it is with sleep. If we are worried, or feeling critical, controlling, depressed, guilty or ashamed, we won't benefit from whatever sleep we manage to have. The key to resolving poor sleep patterns and to achieving better quality of sleep is preparation. Our unconscious "soul" wants resolution and our sleeping body cannot deny this urge. In sleep Vata, Pitta and Kapha are brought up against the emotions and events that have affected us.

Ritual and ceremony help to establish the ideal circumstances for sleep. Within the rhythmic cycle of a day there are periods of stimulation, periods of activity and periods when stimulation should be reduced. This reduction in external sources of stimulation should precede sleep. Awareness is a quality that applies here as much as when extending the capacity of our senses, the difference being that awareness prior to sleep should be directed towards a questioning of our reactions to the outside world and an increase in our response to the inner self.

Deepak Chopra believes that the rituals associated with sleep are the most direct and intimate ways in which we prepare to connect with the inner world. For him the most effective ways to leave the conscious world is to recap the events of our day. We should go through the day, examine our mistakes and the times when we have been out of alignment; we should look at the issues, the moments of lethargy or indecision and the successes, make any apologies that may be necessary (to oneself) and finish with a prayer of gratitude for the day and a request for guidance.

There are other more familiar rituals that are no less important. These rituals are practical processes that involve specific drinks, clothing, scents or aromas, temperature of the bedroom, bedding and bed linen, control of light and the size and nature of our beds. The age old hair brushing ritual adopted by women (100 long, slow brushstrokes before bed) may not only have improved hair condition, but also acted as a powerful signal to the body to prepare for sleep. We may not all have enough hair to warrant that activity, but there are many other simple steps we can follow to take our conscious mind and body into the realm of sleep. All cleansing rituals are important, and washing with a different soap from our usual daytime soap, one that still suits our dosha, but which calms our senses, gives a clear sensual signal. Self-massage or foot massage are similarly powerful ways to attune our minds and bodies to sleep and relaxation. Chanting mantras in a sacred space, with a lighted candle or burning incense, acts on our spiritual sense as does applying essential oils to our pillow.

When we are balanced, sleep is not a problem. It is only when we are out of tune with our doshas that disturbances become significant. In the west we generally neglect the requirements of our sleeping selves and we only pay attention when things aren't going well. Problems with sleep take many forms that are closely related to our doshas. Vata types suffering from insomnia or disturbed sleep patterns are likely to default to the characteristically Vata state of worry and indecision. Whatever has gone on in the day or week will be always be a source of anxiety. They are light sleepers, sensitive to noise and they remember their dreams. Pitta types suffering from disturbed sleep, fall asleep initially more easily than Vata types, but then wake up disturbed. A Pitta imbalance will create overheating, hunger or anger. Things may not have gone the way they wanted or they will suffer from a nagging sense of aggravation or the need to control things and lose sleep accordingly. They too remember their dreams. Sleep disturbances take a different form for Kapha types. They typically fall into a dead sleep for the duration of the night, but wake up unrefreshed. The disturbance to them is deeply felt, without obvious cause. They "die" completely in sleep and will not awaken easily even for noise. They don't remember dreams.

When we are balanced and in harmony with our dosha and life around us we sleep properly. When we fall out of balance our sleep usually suffers. By now you will be more aware of your dosha and its characteristics. In Chapter 9 we will examine imbalances in detail, but in this chapter it is worth pointing out how sleep disturbances and dreams can indicate dosha imbalances in a very direct way. You simply have to practise awareness in recognising what is going on and learn from the immediate experience of a sleep disturbance. Our subconscious wants us to resolve issues or examine problems and it sends messages that keep us awake. When you lie awake, unable to sleep, or if you wake in the night, what is actually happening? Ask yourself what is inside that wants to be out; what have you not examined? For instance, very often there is a guilt component to insomnia. When we lie awake it's frequently because we haven't claimed or recognised an emotion and we are thus given messages to examine particular issues. We need to deal with these issues directly to achieve good quality sleep.

Sleep problems need addressing when they happen, regardless of the time. At those moments we need to take ten minutes to ask ourselves "How does being awake feel—what emotion am I feeling?" We need to see and feel the difference between angst and generalised worry, between nagging, habitual anxiety and heated anger. It may be tiring or uncomfortable to wake oneself enough to ask these questions, but it is worth the effort to solve what can become a debilitating problem if left unattended.

Vata types can more easily resolve anxiety and tension through ritual. They worry more on a general everyday level and benefit more immediately from the levelling, regulating nature of structured, consistent evening routine.

Pitta types suffer from inner angst that ritual alone will not dissolve except for a short time. They need to address issues directly, even in the middle of the night. Pitta types are more likely to work through and resolve their issues through their dreams.

Kapha types have been described as being able to sleep on a clothes line, but unbalanced Kapha sleep is not rejuvenative. Emotions are more likely to be to the fore with Vata and Pitta types, but buried deep in Kapha types and in sleep this is expressed through unconsciousness. They are more able to suppress the underlying emotion and troubling experiences of life they don't want to face, but at the price of a barren experience of the inner world of dreams and healthy sleep.

It's worth examining Kapha sleep in comparison with the two other doshas, since we can learn something about ourselves from this. Vata and Pitta types are more likely to experience emotions openly and express themselves in their individual ways, balanced and imbalanced. Kapha types have a strong tendency to revert to introversion or apathy when imbalanced, and this is reflected in the nature of their sleep and its consequences. It is arguable that imbalanced Kapha types may experience more emotional problems than the other two doshas because of this. The deadness of poor quality Kapha sleep denies them the opportunity to work through issues in dreams in the way that Vata and Pitta types do. This deadness is a denial of emotions, unalleviated by rejuvenation in sleep. They wake up fatigued and even more tired, unable to face things again, the sense of closure spiralling into all aspects of their life. These inner emotions, denied full expression, become visible as physical thickness. Here is where the Kapha tendency to excess weight and immovability originates. Kapha emotions may begin to seep out into anger, unmediated by dreams, and manifested as awkwardness, or as displacement activity such as false laughter, greedy eating habits or gross fingernail biting.

It is interesting to see this disparity between disturbed sleep and expressed emotion in Vata and Pitta types and unexpressed emotion and deadening sleep in Kapha types. These sleep disturbances, which have dosha-like characteristics, can be experienced by the other doshas, so that a Vata type may suffer from Kapha deadness, a Pitta type from Vata anxiety, etc. Chapter 9 will cover other transferred imbalances.

Relaxation

Our minds need respite from thinking in the same way that our bodies need to recuperate from exercise. They need to be helped to stop all activity for certain periods and they need to re-focus through different processes. Meditation has been mentioned a number of times in this book as one of the prime tools for developing inner stability and many other sources of holistic health also recommend it. The daily ritual of meditation is vital to mental recovery, like defragging your computer. Its benefits cross dosha boundaries.

Exercise is similarly beneficial to all doshas, but here differing requirements emerge. Exercise for relaxation differs slightly from exercise for sporting purposes. We need physical activity to maintain our capacity to move, work and function as complex organisms. Our hearts, muscles and lungs benefit from aerobic activity and we develop and enhance co-ordination and motor skills, together with the facility to resist degenerative conditions through weight bearing activity, which also build muscles and the quality of robustness. Weight bearing activity is particularly beneficial to menopausal women. However, one of the main aims of exercise and an important one in relation to relaxation, is the goal of balancing our mind and body. Through exercise we link our physical and spiritual selves. Deepak Chopra points out that exercise, in Ayurvedic terms, should not be work. It is a means to an end, and that end is to be happy, comfortable and prepared for work. Being happy involves avoiding the tedium of punishing routines that only create stress and it involves working to no more than 50% of our capacity. We need to be aware of our heart rate and work within our individual capacity, not pushing things to extremes. And we need to balance the range of our activity. Too much of anything reduces its benefits, and variations in our chosen activity are positively beneficial, refreshing muscles and the nervous system through change and variety. Note that as we age, Vata increases in our bodies and is exacerbated by over-exertion. It is important to recognise this in any exercise programme and we should reduce the intensity of our physical activity accordingly.

The dosha characteristics all come into play within exercise. **Vata's** qualities of movement and change, aid the development and maintenance of agility and co-ordination. **Pitta's** qualities of fire and transformation create circulation and transportation of oxygen and energy around the body. **Kapha's** quality of grounded earthiness creates strength, stability and energy. We all have these doshas within us and they form the foundation upon which all physical activity is undertaken. Our bodies cannot function without the combination of their qualities and our choice of physical activity, which should suit our principal dosha, nevertheless involves all of these qualities.

The particular bias of our principal dosha means that we are better suited to certain ranges of physical activity and in a balanced Ayurvedic lifestyle, our spiritual and physical regimes would compliment one another. Each dosha's exercise and relaxation requirements reflect the things we have already learned. Vata types need to be structured and consolidated; Pitta types need to be cooled and unwound; and Kapha types need to be inspired and rejuvenated.

Walking forms the ideal foundation activity for all doshas, since is creates the best conditions for relaxation, structured movement and controlled pace and stimulation. We have become far too reliant on cars and other forms of transport, and very few people walk far enough on a regular basis. Mountain walking and lots of related activities such as rock climbing, scrambling, fell running, etc., have grown in popularity, and the "Outdoor Scene" thrives in Europe and America, all of which is fine, but is separate from daily life. It is an escape. What's missing is the daily ritual, the mental discipline and the stillness that comes from a regular routine of thirty to sixty minute walks. These daily walks are a perfect foundation for every other spiritual and physical activity we undertake. All doshas also benefit from dance for its rhythmic and structured qualities and its capacity to extend us gently.

Vata types also benefit from Tai Chi and Bhakti Yoga. They do not respond well to over-exertion, but are better suited to structured, consistent activity. They are less suited to cold weather activities unless very well wrapped up. Golf's pace and patterns are good for Vata types. Yoga is best practiced by Vata types with still sitting positions. Deep breathing will help to calm this nervous body and mind.

Type of meditation: Vata types should meditate any time and anywhere, as this dosha will always benefit from being quiet in short bursts. Silent walking meditation where they can be slow and attentive is good for them. Mantras for Vata contain thoughts and words connected to nature, and both meditation and mantra's can be done in natural locations. They should contemplate the universe, God, nature and anything that does not create worry or anxiety. The greatest relaxation practice for Vata is the concept of quiet devotion.

Overall, walking and swimming is good for Vata, but it is important to be warm and comfortable without undertaking strenuous activity.

Pitta types benefit from jogging as well as walking, Hatha Yoga and from more demanding scrambling or mountain climbing. When practising Yoga, sitting and structured positions are best. Deep breathing calms the body and mind and releases aggravation.

In relaxation, meditation is also good for Pitta at any time or place and helps to calm the heated mind. Visualisations of cooling waters and cooling scenes are helpful. So is walking in cool environments, nature, woods, lakesides and streams, all without strain or sustained action. Mantras for Pitta are about removing hostility and creating compassion and peace.

They do not benefit so much from competitive sport because they are already heated and competition simply increases that quality. Swimming is an ideal Pitta activity and Pitta types respond well to winter sport, since their innate heat helps them cope with the cold.

Overall—walking in quiet places alongside water or in the cool evening air in the moonlight is good. Tending gardens and encouraging the growth of fragrant flowers is also good. Many Pittas choose to do hard exercise and this is not good; moderate exercise is much better for Pittas and walking is really beneficial.

Kapha types cope with heavy exercise, weight training and endurance sports. They have the capacity for sustained output of strength. Dancing is good for Kapha types, because grace and improved skill in movement enhances their sense of self. They too, like Vatas, are less well-suited to cold weather activity.

Kapha types can practise Yoga with strong active workouts and standing positions. Meditation on removing greed, possessiveness and attachment is required and with regular karma yoga which depends on active service to others or the community. Mantras should be stimulating with a clearing sound and with active movement.

Overall—Kapha types should be active and do strong aerobic workouts, and they should spend time in the sun and warm windy weather to clear out the 'cobwebs.' They can remain active later in the day than the other doshas. They should avoid having naps during the day, which they often like to do. They should read stimulating books on action and challenging subjects. Travel is excellent for Kapha as it stimulates body and mind. They should avoid cold, damp places and environments.

Gardening or being closely involved with nature at an immediate local level is recommended for all types and here interesting differences come into play. Vata types are suited to looking after or being near large lawns, with the ritual of mowing being of especial benefit to their straying minds. Pitta types benefit from the whole array of natural elements, but especially water features. Kapha types benefit most from variety, details, potted plants and herb gardens.

Reading, music, cultural pursuits and vacations come within the realm of relaxation and here the differing characteristics of each dosha also come into play.

Locations

Sun, sea, sand and exotic places are great for all types provided that consideration is given to the potentially unbalancing factors of heat, dryness and breeziness. When balanced, each dosha can cope with all conditions, and variety is good for all types—the spice of life, in fact. The upsets only occur when a dosha is unbalanced, and when environmental factors exacerbate inherent characteristics.

Vata types don't cope with hot places very well. Holidays are better taken in temperate climates, and in places where dryness is not excessive. Holidays that take them close to or within landscapes, forests, rivers and the sea are preferred. If they find themselves in hot, dry places, they need to maintain hydration, use sunhats, sunglasses and sunscreen and be conscious of their own metabolic response to the heat. They need regularity and calming experiences, with the opportunity for reflection. The colours of sea, sky and mountains in themselves are great for them.

Vata types are naturally creative and responsive to stimulation and planning and organisation best ground this tendency. Within cultural contexts, relaxation can be taken from visits to places of architectural interest, the great cathedrals, bridges, engineering masterpieces and achievements from history and more recent times. They can use the structure, stability and sense of order created by these environments to encourage that quality to grow within themselves. They should not be looking for excessive contrast or sudden juxtaposition of elements, but for continuity and a levelling effect. The sensation of space and the inherently static qualities that pervades grand civic places are wonderful influences on them and such experiences should be planned and scheduled, since Vata types are prone to needing change sooner that Pitta or Kapha types, even within these beneficial arenas.

Vata types are nourished by the narrative flow and structure of films and novels, by the layout and progression of exhibitions of all kinds, and by the form and structure of music. Vata types may only hear the words in songs as sounds that compliment the instrumental backing and, with music as well as the visual arts, they are refreshed by the linear and tonal structure, and by complimentary patterns and combinations.

Pitta types, like Vatas, do not cope with hot places very well, but for a different reason. They are hot and don't need any more heat. They get most out of being on or near water, landscapes and sources of tranquil energy. Like Vata, the colours of sea, sky and mountains are positively uplifting for them. That is not to say they should only go to such places, rather they should balance the range of their recreational experiences.

Pitta's quality of action and transformation gains renewal from contemplation, whether in nature or in the great spiritual places such as cathedrals and inspirational civic spaces. Pitta types can be driven to achieve for too much of their time and benefit from experiences that contain no direct competitive challenge. Cultural experiences that allow them to absorb the influences of cooling sights, sounds and smells are what they need. Direct experience and study of contexts, of the relationship between past and present, and of the relative qualities and nature of life in different cultures, renews a Pitta's inquisitive, organising mind without challenge.

Pitta types like to understand the meaning behind events. They absorb and process information thoroughly and gain from any chance to relieve this processing power and relax into the moment without the need to create action. They benefit from the opportunity to simply experience film, art and music without stress. They gain most from stillness of mind and body.

Kapha types relax best by raising their energy levels, not from contemplation and stillness. This is not to say that meditation and other spiritual practices should be out of Kapha's domain, rather that their minds and bodies also benefit from reinvigorating physical and mental activity. They suit the heat and can enjoy the sun with ease. Hot temperatures and colours enliven their Kapha stillness. The bazaars, the energy and tension within busy streets and alleys, and the constant physical and visual movement of strange and exotic places are great for them, and if such venues are too far away for now, bustling city life, full of colour and contrast and closer to home is equally good.

They re-energise and relax better through movement and activity that can be fairly vigorous, either directly, in the form of immediate action, or indirectly as a spectator. Taking part in or watching competitive sports, seeing action in films, reading about and moving through lively cultural landscapes are all great ways for Kapha types to relax. Whereas Vata and Pitta types gain most from the abstract spiritual experiences of space, landscape and architecture, Kapha types benefit from direct involvement with the bustle and sensory experience of life.

Kapha types relax best by shifting their inherent stillness through direct movement, by observing dynamic movement in nature and by being in the presence of powerful contrasts of sight, sound and smell. They are rested through the experience of movement.

Chapter 7

Combination Doshas

The subject of combination doshas seems to excite most people. By now you will have completed your questionnaire and 99% of you will have realised that you are a combination of all three doshas and your scores for two of them will have been close. You will have been uncertain about many physical and emotional characteristics and you will have been grateful for the opinions of family and friends to help sort out the confusion. Awareness of who and what we are takes time, and the background knowledge you have now begun to assimilate will stand you in good stead for the rest of your life. You are learning about how you fit into the broader environment, about the forces that shaped you and continue to affect your life on a daily, monthly and yearly basis. But you will also see that whilst you may be closer to realising what physical qualities you possess, your emotional qualities may be less clear, and will most likely fluctuate. This is perfectly normal. We are all affected by the events and disturbances of life and our dosha's inherent characteristics mean that we respond in particular ways—always. When we share traits from two doshas, as most of us do, then those responses will come from these shared qualities and we must learn how the ebb and flow of life exacerbates each dosha in turn. We will examine imbalances in Chapter 9, and the effects of the seasons are covered in Chapter 8. For now it is important to get a clearer understanding of our combination dosha so that we can then accommodate these influences according to our type.

It is critical to understand that we all consist of varying quantities of something much larger than ourselves. Each of us consists of all the five elements. These elements remain in a state of dynamic tension within us. We are born with a physical dosha that is unchanging throughout our lives. This is subject to external and internal influences, but we have essentially the same physical constitution we were born with. Weight gain or loss, upsets and upheavals all have their effects but according to Ayurveda we don't change. Knowing what we are and working with this knowledge brings optimal health. When we are a combination of two main doshas, we simply have to work with the different factors relating to each. Emotional and spiritual imbalances will affect our physical body, but we have to see beyond these effects and work with our core being.

Our case studies have been of three individuals who have had their dominant doshas examined for the sake of clarity. It is possible that some people are predominantly one dosha, but they are few and far between. Most of us have a slightly dominant dosha, followed by a secondary dosha, with the third some way back on the scale, and this is the case with Victor, Penelope and Karen, as it is with you. Many people become too hung up on establishing their precise dosha qualities at the first try. We have worked with students and clients who have become so controlling and rigid over their idea of a dosha that they became prisoners of an opinion that removed spontaneity and the joy of discovery from their lives. Don't fall into that trap. Work with what you have learned for now and allow observations, insights and the results of your own experiences to reveal the nuances of your own constitution. Physically you will combine portions of all three doshas, but if you look back to younger days, when you were less affected by time and tide, you will be able to see through the immediate layers of physicality and narrow your dosha down to two main sets of traits at most. Think about the trends and patterns that dominate your emotional responses to life. Again, these will form a fairly consistent pattern that most likely overlaps two doshas. One of these, in each case will eventually be seen to dominate. Don't rush to make a decisive result. Live and grow into awareness of what you really are.

By now you will have experienced tastes and the other senses in a new way. Reading about the case studies and reflecting upon your own experiences will have raised your awareness and you will be seeing dominant traits. Remember that in general terms Vata is concerned with wind and movement, Pitta with fire and heat, and Kapha with earth and stability. How do you feel about these qualities within yourself? Where there is doubt, allow two qualities to come to the fore and work with them. There should be no trauma associated with getting your dosha "right first time". Establish what you think you are now as a guide and work from that.

Here are some examples of people who were initially confused about their dosha.

After working through books and questionnaires Debbie thought she was Vata followed by Pitta. She had looked at her body type and her mental and emotional activity. She worked to balance this Vata element through nutrition and the senses and as she did so the Pitta element became more obvious and pronounced. She began to see that Pitta was her dominant type, with Vata close by and Kapha some way behind. To begin with she was out of balance with both doshas. When you aren't sure about yourself, you are likely to be the same as Debbie with two doshas close together and an imbalance with both. For Debbie, working with one brought the other into play and she could recognise her dominant dosha.

Greta was a large woman with a round smiley face. She worked through the questionnaire and decided she was Pitta. Like many people, she preferred the qualities of one dosha to another, and in this case didn't want to acknowledge her earthy qualities, choosing instead to see what she thought were more desirable Pitta traits. She wanted to be "the leader", and ignored her obvious size and tendency to gain weight. She actually persuaded herself that she had "only just put on weight" and was really much slimmer, despite photographic evidence to the contrary going back to her younger years. She was not obese, simply a large woman, big-boned, tall and strong. Linda found that Greta was in denial, and helped her recognise her true qualities. Like most of us she had two strong metabolic components; she was Kapha with Pitta close behind.

How did this all come to light? Greta believed she was Pitta and ate accordingly. She cut out fire foods, ate earth foods and became tired and lethargic, gaining weight and losing energy. She started to think that Ayurveda didn't work but luckily had a private consultation with Linda. They discovered that she had some Pitta traits—a tendency to be critical, even to herself, and angry— "What's wrong with the weight gain—I'm doing everything I can for my Pitta body type?" and she even started to blame Linda for giving the wrong advice. However the more aware she became, the more obvious her mistake was. Linda encouraged her to re-examine photographs of her younger self. She encouraged Greta to examine her hands, feet and joints. All the evidence was there; it simply needed a shift on Greta's part to see that she had always been a tall, well-balanced and big-boned woman. Even when younger she had never been skinny, but someone who was often described as handsome or "bonny." Her hands and feet were quite large, often a Kapha trait, and when she examined her face she had languid, watery eyes, not the piercing gaze of a typical Pitta. Her sleep patterns were Kapha: she slept heavily and was often not refreshed afterwards. With careful prodding she admitted to snacking between meals and ate sweet things when upset or stressed. She was also unwilling to face up to conflict. All in all, she had more Kapha than Pitta traits.

Greta is a great lesson to many of us. When working through your questionnaire, if you are even slightly overweight, ask a friend to help you. Denial is a Kapha trait yet there is simply no point is ignoring the desirable Kapha characteristics. Greta's qualities of stability, strength and unflappability were major assets in her work and her family life, yet she wanted to deny them in favour of what she at first perceived to be more acceptable characteristics. Many Kapha people do this. The planet is actually short of Kapha structure and strength, so be sure you don't fall into the denial trap if you are a borderline Kapha.

Once Linda had helped Greta to recognise her Kapha/Pitta combination she was able to eat Pitta and Vata tastes, cut down on Kapha food, lose some weight and gain more vitality. Because Pitta was strong in Greta she needed to avoid eating too much in the way of fire foods and a Vata diet would introduce lightness and air into her metabolism. Like Greta, once you have established which combination you are, always work with your strongest dosha.

Going back to Debbie, her Pitta/Vata combination meant she should always be careful of an excess of fire foods. They would always disrupt her Pitta side. Since Pitta and Vata are both "light," an increase in Kapha food would balance both her doshas. She would achieve this not with highly spiced stews and soups, but through eating moderately spicy food, full of earthy root vegetables, and the sweet, sour and salty tastes, with some pungency and astringency. If she found her Vata traits were beginning to rise and dominate, she could then reduce pungent, bitter and astringent tastes.

So, after working through the questionnaires, reading this chapter and still being unsure of which dosha is dominant because they are so close, what do you do now?

You close you eyes and quietly ask yourself these questions:

> Am I hotter or colder?
> Am I more likely to be angry, worried or not bothered?
> Am I more argumentative or more self-critical?

Simple questions can often be the most difficult to answer, so be clear—answer instinctively. For instance, do you prefer cool cotton sheets even in winter, or do you like the bed to be warm to the touch? When someone asks a question do you snap your answer back at them and finish their sentences? Do you make up your mind then change it time and again and ask others for advice? Or are you more likely to sulk and withdraw even in a minor conflict? When you feel low do you worry and blame yourself, do you blame all and everything around you, or do you raid the fridge?

These intuitive questions are important. When you have answered them ask yourself:

> Am I Vata or Pitta?
> Am I Pitta or Kapha?

Let's look at the combination dosha scenario where we've made choices for what is now realised to be the wrong one. Greta had decorated her house to suit a Pitta dosha. The colour scheme was soothing and earthy, designed to cool what she believed to be her excessive Pitta heat. But she often felt tired and lethargic when at home. She loved the décor and the colour scheme but never felt re-energised by time at home. Her dominant Kapha dosha, with its earthy, slow moving quality, was actually being thrown out of balance by the preponderance of earth themes and colours at home. This wasn't a problem. She didn't need to redecorate, simply to adapt. Linda advised Greta to buy fresh flowers and live plants with vibrant Kapha-focussed colours, and to accessorise the house with brightly coloured, lively looking cushions and throws. She could bring in a sense of movement with textures and contrasts of shape and scale. The beige settees could have colourful scatter cushions, and interesting cameos could be created to stimulate the eye. She wasn't introducing clutter but she was creating the stimulation a Kapha type needed.

Eventually this situation improved. Earth colours would calm Greta's secondary Pitta dosha, but her dominant Kapha dosha required more attention. Had the situation been reversed, so that Pitta dominated, there would still have been no problem. An interior that was too hot could have been toned down to create cooler tones, and more space. One wall could have been cool and the other hot without creating too much Pitta stimulation, and accessories and details could have been simplified, with cooling Pitta colours to soothe that dosha.

With combination doshas, even though the body types may be mixed, we are still more likely to be one than another and we can deal with that relatively easily, as our examples show. We make our assessments, work on that basis and monitor our reactions. Our emotions are also likely to be out of sync and it is important to realise that the emotional side to our dosha is continually bombarded by external and environmental influences, so confusion is inevitable at first. Take heart, because when we get our bodies into a more balanced state everything else tends to follow.

There are various opinions on the possible number of dosha combinations. Some authorities believe there are nine possible combinations, others believe there are seven. Some texts claim that some people are evenly tri-dosha. In our opinion we all have Vata, Pitta and Kapha within us and it is impossible to be only one dosha. It is inevitable that one of the combinations will arise in the body. If, however, you believe yourself to be a single dosha type and work only to balance that dosha, it is likely that other traits and qualities will emerge from the other two. You will then have to deal with them, otherwise a series of imbalances will erupt. We think that the most likely scenario for those who think they are a single dosha is that one dosha may dominate for most of the time, but the others are still there in the background.

A typical family will contain different dosha combinations. If there are real imbalances with high stress levels or illness, it is most advisable to understand that individual's doshas and treat them separately, with special nutritional and environmental considerations being taken into account. As long as the group is not excessively out of balance there are no real problems in coping with the needs of different doshas. **It is best to eat fresh seasonal food that includes all six tastes every day**. Over the course of a day all six tastes can be covered and remember that the pungent, bitter and astringent tastes are really accents that can come from the addition of herbs and spices and that too much can be bad for any dosha.

In the family context it is important to examine the tastes (see Chapter 3). Meals based on fresh seasonal food can easily have accents added to suit each family member and simple changes are highly effective. Individual needs can be accommodated by adding accents of the necessary taste to a core menu and reducing the tastes that aggravate. As a general principle:

- Vata can add more salt and cut down on cups of tea and coffee (astringent);

- Pitta can take in extra sweetness by adding fennel or creamy sauces and should have no extra salt and cut down on alcohol;

- Kapha should add hot and peppery spices and leave out the creamy sauces, gravy and vinegar-based dressings.

The seasonal extremes of summer and winter appear at first to present the greatest possibility for conflict, but in reality there are no serious problems.

In summer, when all the family wants salads:

- Vata types need not be left out; they should add thick creamy mayonnaise and boiled new/salad potatoes.

- Pitta should add fresh apple and a light coconut-based dressing, or cooler dressings using sunflower or coconut oil.

- Kapha can eat twice the amount of lettuce and greens and add oil-free lemon dressing.

In winter, when everyone wants heartening stews:

- Vata can add dumplings and extra salt.
- Pitta can leave out the salt and sprinkle on ground fennel instead, and enjoy the dumplings.
- Kapha can leave out the dumplings and extra salt, hold back on the potatoes, double the vegetable content and add a chilli dressing to their own portion.

These examples should help you to apply commonsense and the principles of the six tastes and doshas to family mealtimes.

Chapter 8

The Seasons

The seasonal cycle is one of the most tangible examples we could have of being a part of a much greater living organism. Seasonal change and weather conditions profoundly affect all life on the planet, governing the growth of plant life (and thus animal life) and also the changing conditions of our global environment and the more immediate local surroundings that we live in. Sunlight, temperature, humidity and rainfall in varying combinations form the basis for suitable living conditions for most life forms on the planet and our societies were founded on the availability of food in the locations we chose to live in. Our metabolisms are keyed into our local environment. Planes, trains and road transport can now bring us food from all over the world at all times of the year but we still cannot cheat the seasons. Eating mangoes in Northern Europe during winter doesn't make it summertime! The seasons unfold in an endless sequence on a global scale and we live through that continually changing context.

Each season's climatic changes produce distinct shifts in our metabolism on a cyclical basis. The changes are good for our bodies because they provide opportunities for rebuilding and growth. The winter months are periods of recuperation from the gradually increasing dryness and heat of the summer months, when our bodies become depleted by hot sun, hot air movement and the acidity, astringency and pungency created by months of harsh sunlight which sucks nutrients and evaporates water from the soil, even in the more temperate climate of the UK, when cloud cover is more frequent than blue skies. We associate summer with holidays and excitement, and indeed it can be the perfect season for all kinds of activities. Crops are harvested and long summer days are beautiful to experience. Nevertheless, summer heat saps energy and depletes our reserves, which is why despite our love of the weather we sit in the shade, plaster ourselves in sunscreen and drink lots of fluids. In winter we gain strength and substance from the damper conditions, the slowing down of our metabolism and a gradual increase in the earth's water levels.

Not the balance of attributes some people might expect, but that is the reality; we recuperate and gain strength throughout winter and expend that strength and energy during the summer. The seasons are our earth's expression of the full range of dosha characteristics, and so there are Vata, Pitta and Kapha periods of the year, which aggravate our own doshas. Seasonal change is good when our lives are settled, but stressful during periods of transition; and there are two critical junctures (occurring around November 22 to December 9 and June 8 to 24) when our health is severely at risk and when vigilance is needed. These two junctures are the periods when we should organise our physical and emotional resources in preparation for the rigours of seasonal changes, which can have severe weakening effects on our wellbeing. Although, due to the ease of importation, we can now buy food from anywhere in the world, it is better to stick to the seasonal foods of the country we live in and to use imported, out of season food as treats, We need to allow our bodies to go through the seasonal changes that affect our immediate environment and to nurture them with food that corresponds with those seasons. The seasons create demands on our bodies that can only be met by responding with seasonally appropriate nutrition and activity. We need to live sympathetically with cycles of seasonal change, which are as central to being alive as any other sensory experience. That means learning to work with the six tastes on a day-to-day basis and learning to balance the phases of our activity over longer periods of time. The rewards are vigour, health and strength and pleasure arising from harmony rather than struggle.

Many people are confused by the cause of the seasons and some believe they occur because the earth moves away from the sun. This is not true. Our planet experiences seasonal variations because it moves in two distinct ways. It spins in a balanced consistent manner and it orbits around the sun. The controlled spin occurs around what is known as an axis, rather like the centre of a spinning top. This axis is tilted and the tilt means that at different times of the year the northern and southern hemispheres each receive longer and shorter periods of sunlight. We will explain this in detail in the coming paragraphs and in diagrams in Appendix G. Note that the earth's orbit does not affect the seasons, since it is practically a circular orbit, and to all intents and purposes the earth remains a constant distance from the sun. However, the earth's axis *is* tilted and this creates the varying lengths of night and day and a significant variation in the qualities of the seasons.

The earth is a huge spherical mass that rotates around a central axis once every 24 hours. The axis is best imagined as a knitting needle pushed through the central core of a huge apple. This creates a North Pole and a South Pole, an Arctic and an Antarctic. If we hold the needle upright (vertical) and rotate it the apple revolves in exactly the same way that the earth rotates and we can imagine or even mark a line around the widest part. This is the equator, a line that divides the planet into a top half and a bottom half or a Northern and a Southern Hemisphere. The equator is also known as the line of zero degrees latitude. Other lines of latitude also run around the world, parallel to the equator and going gradually nearer to the poles. They are known as the high latitudes. Imagine the effects of sunlight shining towards this homemade planet. The rotation brings the planet into and then out of alignment with the sun, creating periods of sunlight and darkness.

Look at the curve of your apple-earth. You can see how certain parts of the surface are more directly in line with the sun—these aren't curving away towards the poles and therefore would receive more direct sunlight and consequently hotter conditions. That is why the seas and countries nearer the equator are the hottest part of the planet. The sun is high overhead, creating more heat. Now look toward the poles. The sun's rays hit the apple-earth's surface at a much less direct angle; because of this there is less heat and the areas nearer the poles, the high latitudes, become progressively colder the nearer we get to each pole. This corresponds with what we know: Africa and Asia, the Caribbean and the Mediterranean and parts of North and South America are very hot and it gets colder up north, or in the far south. When the sun gets lower in the sky towards sunset, light levels drop and these lower light levels would be the norm at the two poles all year round because sunlight would always be at a very low angle. If things remained the way they are on your home-built apple-earth, with the axis and the two poles completely vertical, then the seasons would be fixed. It would always be summer in some parts of the world around the equator and always winter in other regions that were progressively closer to the poles. There would always be either light and heat, or darkness and cold, but we know that this isn't so. Everywhere on earth experiences both a summer and a winter, even in the Arctic and the Antarctic. What we know from experience is that the closer a location is to the Equator, the more even the balance is between daylight and darkness, not varying much from twelve hours of each every day of the year.

Why are there seasonal variations in sunlight? To understand this let's go onto the last stage. You are still holding the apple-earth and you need to choose an object in the middle of the room to represent the sun (a table or chair). Tilt the top of the needle to towards the imaginary sun (the earth's axis is tilted to 23.5 degrees). You can see how the northern hemisphere now receives more sunlight than the southern and also how the sun's most direct rays have shifted slightly from the equator to another region. You can also see that sunlight now reaches as far as the North Pole. Make a mark on the surface most directly in line with the sun and rotate your apple-earth (without altering the tilt of the axis). You will create the effect of day turning into night as the point you have marked passes from the light into darkness and back in to the light again. This rotation is the equivalent of our 24-hour circadian cycle. The tilt directly towards the sun has created high summer in the Northern Hemisphere, with 24-hour daylight at the North Pole. This is the longest day of the year throughout the Northern Hemisphere, with the greatest amount of sunlight, and known as the Summer Solstice or Midsummer's day, on June 21 or 22.

If you look at your apple-planet at this point you can see that the sun is not directly above the equator but at a slightly higher latitude, marking the position of another circle around the earth, parallel to and north of the equator. This line of latitude is known as the Tropic of Cancer and it marks the farthest point north on the earth's surface at which the sun will be directly overhead. Look again and you will see that in the Southern Hemisphere you have created winter, as the South Pole receives no sunlight despite the daily rotation of your apple-earth. This is the Southern Hemisphere Winter Solstice. Now cross the room to a point directly opposite where you started from without altering the tilt of your earth's axis. As you cross the room the tilt of the axis will take the "North Pole" away from the sun and bring the "South Pole" towards the sun. It is now winter in the Northern Hemisphere when we have the shortest day, known as Midwinter, or the Winter Solstice on December 21 or 22. At the same time it is summer in the Southern Hemisphere, Midsummer's day in fact! The sun is once again not above the equator but this time south of it, marking the other great circle of latitude known as the Tropic of Capricorn.

You have walked your planet from one seasonal extreme to another, and that represents six months of real time on earth. Our planet achieves this change because it orbits around the sun over a period of 365 days and the seasonal range from summer to the next summer occurs within that timescale. During this cycle there are two other phases known as equinoxes when the earth is midway between the summer and winter solstices and they are also significant. March 20 or 21 is the spring equinox for the Northern Hemisphere, and September 22 or 23 is the autumnal equinox for the Northern Hemisphere (they are reversed for the Southern Hemisphere). These are the mid points of the earth's orbit between the extremes of summer and winter, and at these times every part of the earth has an equal balance of 12 hours of daylight and 12 hours of darkness. We experience changeable weather and greater tidal ranges during these periods.

In summary, the inclination of the earth's axis means that at different locations on its orbit the intensity and duration of sunlight varies. This is what we experience with every day that passes. When the Northern hemisphere is tilted toward the sun, the Northern hemisphere receives the most direct sunlight (that is, the angle of incidence is steeper), and it is summer *in the Northern hemisphere*. If the Southern hemisphere is tilted toward the sun, the Southern hemisphere receives the most direct sunlight and it is summer *in the Southern hemisphere*. In the intermediate situations, halfway between the two extremes, the earth's axis is still tilted, but not tilted *with respect to the sun's rays*, and the sun's rays strike directly on the Equator. If the earth's axis was not tilted, the Equator would always be the part of the earth's surface that was closest to the sun and the two poles would always be the farthest points away from the sun at all times. The two Polar Regions would always be in darkness, and in a perpetual winter.

You can now see how the two kinds of movement, rotation and orbit, create seasonal cycles. The orbit creates gradual transition between seasons but does not lessen the extreme seasonal conditions to which we are exposed. The earth's orbit is not quite circular but slightly elliptical (or oval) and many people wrongly assume that the earth moves close to the sun during an orbit, thus creating seasonal change, but this is not so, as we have demonstrated. The path of this orbit is known as the Plane of the Ecliptic. From our diagram in Appendix G you will see these seasonal distinctions clearly.

The determining factor for the seasonal changes is the average daytime temperature. This depends on the amount of heat that the earth receives in a single day and this is determined by the number of hours the sun is above the horizon and how long it spends at its highest point above the horizon. The sun is at its hottest when it is directly overhead. We know this from our daily experience. In summer the hours around midday are the hottest, when we shelter in the shade, and early morning and evenings are cooler, when the sun angles down towards the horizon. It is warm enough to sit outside but we don't fry in the same heat as in the midday glare. Every square metre on the earth's surface is heated at a rate determined by how directly those rays hit the surface. The higher the sun gets, the less slanted its rays become and the more effectively it heats the surface. The greatest effect is felt where the rays hit the surface at their steepest, most vertical angle. For a tilted earth there are days in the year where this heating effect is at its highest, in summer. At other times the sun never gets very high above the horizon and its heating ability is lower, in winter.

More localised and detailed qualities of heat or cold, dryness and humidity and the precise timing and dates of seasonal change come from our proximity to water, sea currents and surrounding landmasses. For instance, the Gulf Stream, one of the most powerful ocean currents in the world, originates in the warmth of the Gulf of Mexico and flows across the Atlantic, bringing warmth to the UK and northwest Europe. It is the reason we have relatively mild winters. The average annual temperature of northwest Europe is about 9°C above the average for our latitude. Semi-tropical plants grow in parts of north-west Scotland that seem entirely out of place with the harsher northern geography. The warm wet weather we are familiar with helps crops and maintains a reasonable balance between dryness and moistness. In contrast the central landmasses of Europe, Russia and Asia experiences no such mediating effects from warming sea currents and winters are deeper and harsher. North America experiences mostly temperate weather conditions with some extremes: Florida and Hawaii are tropical, Alaska is arctic and the Great Plains are semi-arid. Within vast continents living conditions and seasonal effects are widely varied, requiring high levels of awareness and vigilance on the part of their inhabitants, as we shall see shortly.

The seasons share dosha characteristics with us, hardly surprising since the five elements pervade all life on the planet. Certain periods of the year have very specific Vata, Pitta or Kapha qualities related to the seasonal tendency for moistness, dryness, windy roughness or heat. These are times when we have to be very wary because these seasonal variations are as damaging to us as incorrect nutrition. There are two critical seasonal junctures, in late November and June, when we are at most vulnerable. Within these seasonal tendencies variations come about due to sudden changes in the weather, and we need to pay heed to our dosha's needs with the same attention we have given to other environmental considerations.

The seasons also have characteristics that correspond to the six tastes and it is better to balance our nutrition to what best suits both our dosha and the season. Food and seasonal factors cause an accumulation or increase of dosha characteristics. Cold dry weather and wind accumulate Vata; hot weather and humidity accumulate Pitta; cold and wet weather accumulate Kapha. As these qualities accumulate, they aggravate us and imbalances can develop. We can correct these tendencies with nutrition and activity best suited to our dosha.

In the Northern hemisphere, which includes Europe, North America and Asia, the following sequence of seasonal conditions occurs (the reverse applies to the Southern hemisphere, including Australia and New Zealand). The northern phase of the earth's orbit—when the tilt of the earth's axis places the Northern hemisphere in more direct alignment with the sun and we move from late winter to summer—is a weakening period in the year, when the sun and wind gradually develop a harsh drying effect, draining all life in that hemisphere. This increases the bitter, pungent and astringent tastes, which constrict and absorb moisture, aggravating Vata and Pitta doshas and alleviating Kapha.

The southern phase of our orbit is a period when the tilt of the earth's axis takes us out of direct alignment with the sun, moving from summer through autumn and early winter, creating cloudier and wetter conditions that cool us down, providing the opportunity for growth and recovery. The sweet, sour and salty tastes become dominant, contributing to bulk and power, aggravating Kapha and alleviating Vata and Pitta.

There are many different interpretations of the number of seasons in an Ayurvedic year and in Asia (the continent of its origin) six seasons are recognised, caused by pre- and post-monsoon seasons and other factors that we don't experience in the west. We tend to be preoccupied with our immediate circumstances and think of our year comprising of four seasons—winter, spring, summer, autumn. In the UK these are often thought of as wet, wetter, cold and wet (and wetter still by some!), but when we look at the overall picture finer distinctions do occur. A four-season model might be easier to grasp or work with yet the only real difference from the six seasons described by the early sages, is the rainy season, which we do not experience as a monsoon. Even so, the late summer months are humid in most countries and there are significantly different factors at work in the environment. Late winter may not always feel cool and dewy, in the Asian model, but there is a difference between that period and early winter that we actually feel. The differences work with and against our doshas and are manifested in the food we eat. Whilst immediate seasonal conditions affect us directly (and sometimes it can be hard to distinguish between summer and winter in north European countries) , the sources of our food and the genetic inheritance of seeds which ultimately feed all living creatures have seasonal timescales programmed into their DNA. This inheritance is what nurtures us through the seasons. What goes on at the planetary level is the determining factor for health and our genetic inheritance is fully loaded with rhythms of seasonal change. We should be sensitive to the full range of seasons and eat seasonal food. We will examine seasonal foods in more detail later in this chapter, but we stress that regardless of local variations in climate, seasonal variations are programmed into our cells. The table in Appendix G shows where both sets of seasonal boundaries fall and the two critical seasonal junctures in the year.

During the periods of seasonal change we should be especially careful with the tastes that correspond to our dosha and use them sparingly. Equally, as every season changes we need to take care of a general increase in Vata. **Two critical junctures, one in early winter around November 22 to December 9 and the other in summer around June 8 to 24 are when we are most susceptible to illness and disease.**

The period leading up to the Northern Solstice (summer) is considered to be weakening because the increasing strength of the sun, accompanied by drying winds which gradually drain the earth's energies, dissipates the earth's cool nurturing qualities, increasing levels of the pungent, bitter and astringent tastes and the accompanying qualities of sharpness, dryness and heat. The sun literally burns up life energy, so despite the fact that we love and need summer weather and all that goes with it, this half of the year, the northern phase of our orbit around the sun, is gradually damaging to health without the right kind of preparation and maintenance. We balance the effects of these seasons using sweet, sour and salty tastes.

The three seasons leading up to the Southern Solstice (winter) provide the opportunity to gain strength, when heat and dryness are replaced by moist and cool conditions and we regain the energy depleted by the hotter seasons. Sour, salty and sweet tastes predominate in nature, creating the conditions for growth and the re-building of strength and we use the pungent, bitter and astringent tastes to maintain balance.

Seasonal Eating

The following is a summary of the seasons and the tastes appropriate to each one. Remember that the season to be most careful about is the one that matches your own dosha. That is when you are most liable to upsets and imbalances. **Eat mainly the balancing tastes, not the ones corresponding to your dosha.**

Early winter: mid November—mid January

Eat: warm, heavier food comprising of sweet, sour and salty, tastes, wellcooked and in reasonable quantities, with warm drinks. This is a period of re-building and growth and we need enough food to fuel the changes our bodies undergo.

Avoid: bitter, astringent and pungent tastes and dry, cold and raw foods.

This is a Kapha season when all doshas, especially Vata, need to guard against drafts and dampness.

Late winter: mid January—mid March

If we consider the winter period as a whole there is a shift in emphasis from a Kapha bias with the dominant sweet taste to a Vata bias with a dominant bitter taste. This is a time for consolidation, when our capacity for growth and endurance is built around Kapha qualities. The movement of Vata and trans-formational qualities of Pitta mobilise the resources that come from Kapha sweetness and if these are absent we tend to retreat into our shells and become sluggish and withdrawn. In the winter period Kapha strengthens our immune system and lubricates all tissues, joints and connecting tissues and enhances the power of the digestive system. Winter's contracting quality of cold concentrates *agni*, our digestive fire, and as long as we are healthy we can cope with heavier food in greater quantities. This balances the Vata dosha later in the winter. It is obvious that cold weather is not the time for cold food or drinks, nor is it the time to fast. Warm, cooked grains, soups, proteins, beans and honey and milk should feature in our diet at this time, and any weight gain is perfectly natural as we renew our strength. It is important not to hibernate too much. We should embrace the opportunity winter provides to be quiet and to nurture ourselves, but we should also wrap up against the weather and maintain movement and sufficient levels of activity to overcome the Kapha tendency towards inertia. Late winter's movement towards the bitter taste of Vata dosha is balanced by the earthy tastes of Kapha.

During winter Kapha problems of mucous can occur, and coughs and colds are a common occurrence. When these problems arise we balance them with pungent, bitter and astringent tastes.

Eat: sour, salty, moderately sweet tastes in substantial quantities, with warm food and drink, wellcooked and easily digestible.

Avoid: excessively sweet, pungent and bitter tastes and dry, cold and raw foods. This is essentially a Vata season when that dosha's qualities become aggravated, and when Pitta is balanced.

Spring: mid March—mid May

Spring is when the astringent taste begins to dominate. Kapha accumulated in our bodies over the winter dissolves, creating imbalances such as hay fever, colds and flu—not what we expect with the onset of brighter weather, but that is what happens. The sudden release of Kapha unsettles all life and we balance this with light, bitter and fresh foods, which shift the accumulated Kapha and cleanse our systems. Since we want to move any toxins and excesses that may have built up through winter we avoid heavy, oily, sweet and sour foods.

Eat: pungent, bitter and astringent tastes, moderately sweet, moderately salty warm food in moderate quantities.

Avoid: sweet sour and excessively salty tastes, oily and heavy food, excess fluid and cold food and drink. This is a Kapha season when Kapha diseases can occur in all doshas.

Summer: mid May—mid July

Summer brings heat, dissipation of moisture and resources, and dryness, when the pungent taste of Pitta dominates. The increased heat lowers *agni* and digestive power is impaired. Smaller meals that include sweet, moist, and cool ingredients are best at this time of year, and milk, rice and fruit should feature in our diets. Spicy, hot, pungent, sour and salty foods at this time can irritate the Pitta in all of us, regardless of our main dosha.

Eat: sweet, bitter and astringent tastes, cool food and drinks, and enough fluid to remain hydrated, but not after meals, in order to avoid dousing the digestive fire (agni). It's best to eat some raw or steamed foods, ghee, milk, rice, and saladsbalanced with oils and dressing for Vata types. Maintain good fluid intake, but don't drink after meals, as this inhibits your digestive abilities.

Avoid: sour, salty and pungent tastes, overeating and excessively cold drinks, which affect your ability to digest food. This is a Pitta season so Pitta types especially must avoid the overheating they are naturally prone to in this hottest season.

Late summer/Early Autumn/Rainy Season: mid July—mid September

This is the season that causes the greatest misunderstandings for many people who say that rainy seasons only occur in certain regions close to the tropics. This is true and only relatively few areas of the planet experience genuine monsoon conditions. However, this period is unsettling and often unstable; summer storms, soaring humidity and periods of sultry heat can rapidly change to cool and changeably breezy conditions. This is a difficult time when we may still be recovering from hot summer weather, or still experiencing it, causing unrest in all doshas. Though this is still a Pitta period, local conditions may need monitoring for changes to the dosha character of the prevailing conditions. Soil that has died over the spring and summer can suddenly be saturated by heavy rain, creating greater sourness that affects each dosha even more. This transitional period between the Northern and Southern solstice is when larger planetary forces begin to exert influence on all life.

Late summer/rainy season is dominated by the sour taste and is a period of transition that can aggravate all doshas. Sudden changes between sun and rain, between heat and chill, mean that both Pitta and Vata can be affected at the same time, whilst soil acidity which has been concentrated in the summer heat, is released by rain, affecting Kapha. Honey for sweetness, grains, vegetable soups and a general vigilance and willingness to respond to changes in temperature and humidity with warmer or cooler foods is useful in combating the variability of this time of year.

Eat: sweet, bitter and astringent tastes and cool foods, similar to summer, which do not tax the digestive system. Balance seasonal variability with warmer food and drink and salty tastes to pacify Vata.

Avoid: pungent and sour tastes, cold drinks and excessive activity.

Autumn: mid September—mid November

Autumn is dominated by the salty taste and a transition from Pitta to Vata conditions. The heat of summer and instability of late summer/rainy season shifts to a period of cooler nights and mornings when air and ether elements increase. Vata imbalances such as aching joints and dry skin can increase in all doshas and the Vata tendency towards anxiety is heightened by the imminent seasonal juncture of the late autumnal equinox. Vata types feel the cooler temperatures more keenly than Pitta and Kapha types, but all need to take in moist, warm and well-lubricated foods with sweet, sour and salty tastes.

Eat: sweet, bitter and astringent tastes, easily digestible warmer food in moderate quantities and warm water to flush the system.

Avoid: heavy oily or fatty meals, sour, salty and pungent tastes.

This is a Pitta season, which becomes Vata towards the latter part of the period.

General guidelines with seasonal eating

Eat fresh local food at all times of the year. This will ensure an adequate level of seasonally appropriate food in your diet. The concept of local food has changed with the widespread availability of any kind of food from anywhere in the world at any time of year. The problem with basing a diet on non-local and non-seasonal food is that we aggravate the state of balance that should exist by bringing in, for instance, the pungency of southern hemisphere summer-grown produce into a body living through a northern hemisphere winter. Our core diet should be essentially correct and in line with the season we are living through and to that diet we can add tastes from other seasons and countries as accents. The constant availability of non-seasonal foods in every supermarket undermines our body's location within its own seasonal zone. We need to reinforce our own sense of place and time through our food. Local, in a British context, is best thought of as being from the north or south of the country. In Europe similar geographical divisions can be employed with north/south and east/west being the determining factors. The main criteria are that food that forms our core diet comes from within 500 miles from our home, not another continent.

Each of the six tastes should be present in each meal if possible, but the dominant seasonal taste should be reduced in addition to the normal balancing of tastes that maintain our particular dosha's balanced condition. If our constitutions are balanced then changing environmental factors will have less effect than if we slip out of balance. Vata types can wrap up to keep warm in autumn and winter and also benefit from the cool (not cold), clear, fresh conditions, as long as they are careful during really changeable cold and blustery weather. Pitta types can maintain hydration and avoid excessive sunlight and remain comfortable in hot weather by spending time in the shade, having cool baths and wearing light natural fabrics. Kapha types can avoid the excesses of weight gain, fluid retention and build up of mucous in spring and early summer by having regular daily walks, wearing light natural clothing and eating plenty of dry salads.

The progression of the seasons and their relationship to our doshas are clearly mapped in the table in Appendix G.

Daily Cycle

The seasonal cycle is mirrored by our daily cycle. Over each 24-hour period our bodies undergo six phases of change, experienced in two main cycles, controlled by the sun's light and heat. Beginning with the early hours of dawn, at approximately 6.00 am and going through to sleeping hours just before the next dawn, we go through a sequence of Kapha, Pitta and Vata phases, which repeat in the second cycle beginning at approximately 6.00 pm. These cycles occur irrespective of our own dosha.

The approximate times are:

Dawn:	6.00 am to 10.00 am	Kapha
Morning:	10.00 am to 2.00 pm	Pitta
Afternoon:	2.00 pm to 6.00 pm	Vata
Early evening:	6.00 pm to 10.00 pm	Kapha
Late evening:	10.00 pm to 2.00 am	Pitta
Pre-dawn:	2.00 am to 6.00 am	Vata

Towards the end of sleep Vata's cold, dry mobility is replaced, around dawn, by heavy Kapha energy. We are slow, relaxed after sleep and calm. The morning progresses to a Pitta phase towards noon when we are at our most active and the sun is at its highest. Because this is a Pitta phase our digestive and transformational qualities are at their strongest and our working output and ability to responds physically is at its peak. Our Vata phase follows as the sun loses some of its power. This is the time of maximum mental alertness as a result of Vata's nervous energy. Then the second Kapha phase follows and we slow down and rest. This is the time when we should prepare for bed, but unfortunately many pressures keep us up later than nature intended. The last phases of wakefulness is a Pitta phase, less strong than earlier and one which we should try to avoid by sleeping. In this phase digestion continues and our metabolism is heated as we continue the process of re-building within our bodies. During the night the last Vata phase occurs and, as we have discovered, considerable mental activity takes place including REM sleep. Chapter 6 describes the two systems that control sleep and wakefulness in our bodies and there you can see how our biological clocks operate within the dosha-based cycles that we have just described.

We are meant to rise at dawn and to retire to bed as daylight fades. These are the two ends of a natural daily rhythm that humans have followed for thousands of years and even though life is less governed by available light than it was for our ancestors, we are still made of the same genetic material. The daily and seasonal cycles described here form the underlying template against which our true natures can shine.

Rising early without panic still within a Vata period is best for everyone. Sleeping in too late takes us into the early morning Kapha phase and we never seem to shake off our sleepiness. Between noon and 1.00pm is an ideal time for lunch because it is in the middle of our first Pitta phase when our digestive fire is at its strongest. This is when we should eat the largest meal of the day. The afternoon's activities are fuelled by lunch and our Vata phase allows for creativity and the mental agility to solve problems and finish the working day with tomorrow's tasks clearly defined. (Remember that any afternoon sleepiness is an indication of sleep debt, which is an issue you must resolve by sleeping. Short naps can help but chronic afternoon fatigue is a clear sign that you aren't getting to bed early enough.) The second Kapha phase allows us to slow down, eat what should be a smaller evening meal and establish the calm conditions that should precede sleep. This smaller meal should not tax our digestion, but most people in the west are not used to such an arrangement and eat their largest meal at this time. It is much better to change eating habits and allow our bodies an easier passage through the night with a smaller and lighter digestive load. This is also the period when we should taper off our contact with bright lights and allow the circadian rhythm to take us towards sleep. The reason Ayurveda advocates bedtime before the beginning of the second Pitta phase is that we tend to reawaken as Pitta comes in again and become trapped into wakefulness at the wrong time for our bodies. We may have reset our biological clocks through years of late nights and bright TV and it takes a while for changes to occur, but by reducing the light levels we are exposed to during the late evening hours and by exposing ourselves to daylight in the early morning we can re-establish waking and sleeping rhythms that work with our bodies rather than against them and, critically, which work naturally with the changing seasons that have such a profound effect on all life on the planet.

Chapter 9

Dosha Imbalances

The work described in these final chapters is highly effective in treating common ailments and dealing with the rigours of everyday life, but any severe or chronic conditions require investigation by a qualified Ayurvedic practitioner.

Disturbances are more or less inevitable and can be caused by many things: eating the wrong food, being in the wrong environment, wearing the wrong clothes—these and all the things we have already discussed can aggravate your dosha, but stress at work or within the family, seasonal changes, excessive partying, late nights and lack of sleep, shift work and many other factors can conspire to throw us into imbalanced states.

Many people become confused by the nature and cause of imbalances. They may have learned that they are Vata dosha, for instance, yet begin suffering from the heavy, bloated feelings associated with Kapha. A Pitta type may become agitated and distracted in a Vata fashion and Kapha types may become overheated with Pitta anger. These contrasts to normal healthy sensations may seem confusing, but things become clearer when examined against the context of the Qualities and Attributes (see Appendix H). As we have seen in Chapter 7, whilst we may be predominantly one dosha we all contain aspects of the other doshas. When aggravation crops up in our life, symptoms will emerge from those other facets of our dosha make-up.

Understanding our dosha mix and working with the whole range of attributes brings optimum health. Knowing our primary, secondary and minor doshas allows us to work with the shifting conditions we experience in everyday life. Awareness enables us to anticipate and correct imbalances and it is usually when we lose track of our needs or the circumstances around us that things begin to go wrong and an accumulation of factors can then conspire to throw us off balance. The secret lies in understanding what is behind each occurrence and the key to that deeper level of self-knowledge is found in the qualities.

In Chapter 1 we discussed the qualities specific to each dosha and in Chapter 3 how those same qualities occur in the context of the six tastes. Now we'll look at how they are manifested when we become imbalanced—to do this refer to Appendix H. These qualities form the building blocks of our doshas. If one or more of them becomes excessive then we feel the effects as a discomfort of some kind. When we identify the nature of a discomfort in terms of the qualities we can relieve it using Ayurvedic principles of balance. How? To begin with we always look to our primary dosha and look at the disharmony in the context of how that dosha might manifest an imbalance. The dominant dosha will give a clue. Then we identify the nature of any pain or discomfort when it occurs by referring to the qualities associated with each dosha and asking ourselves if the pain or feeling is hard or soft, piercing or dull, heavy or light, hot or cold and so on through the list of qualities. We might find that the symptoms reflect a quality from our secondary or minor dosha. After identifying the source quality we can begin to address both the cause and the remedy. We will look at this in more detail through our three case studies in the following pages.

The qualities of our primary dosha are nurtured through nutrition, exercise and the balancing activities we have discussed. When these needs are neglected, when we allow other less appropriate factors to impinge on our dosha, then we stop functioning properly. When our sensory input doesn't compliment our main dosha things go wrong. An analogy can be made with a car. If we put petrol in a car with a diesel engine, it won't work. Petrol is a fuel, but it's the wrong fuel. If we try to use the car, the petrol will actually damage the diesel engine. That is an obvious point, but our own imbalances come about precisely because of similar ill-advised activity.

The obvious problem is that family, professional and social pressures, deadlines, travelling conditions and a host of environmental factors conspire to steal our attention from how we are in the moment. Discomfort creeps up and we ignore it until it becomes chronic; rest and sleep are too often looked upon as inconveniences in a busy and crowded lifestyle; food "takes too long to prepare." Suddenly we feel ill or out of sorts but we're not sure why and if we do nothing about it, eventually we become accustomed to feeling unwell. We flounder around wondering why this came about; then many people will pop another pill, have another drink or blast around the gym, or the clubs, or the shopping mall and mask the original problem, which will only re-occur. This is not good, and it can all be avoided, but unless we learn to be specific about the good and the bad sensations, we continue to live in a muddle and things "happen to us." The reality is that the things we do to mask our discomforts are examples of neglectful, self-damaging behaviour. When we strengthen our powers of observation and insight we take control and actually create the life we choose.

Victor, Penelope and Karen are no exceptions to the problems of imbalance, as we have learned. Though they had relieved initial problems they could still be susceptible to seasonal disorders or to the effects of stress. It is quite natural for new factors to emerge that create disturbances, and ongoing chronic stress-inducing issues, such as travel, require continual vigilance. It is difficult to avoid every damaging external influence as we are all susceptible to shifting internal emotional currents. Let's examine the problems they faced as typical Vata, Pitta and Kapha types, with secondary and minor doshas, and what we learn can be applied to your own situation.

Victor is predominantly Vata. In previous chapters we concentrated exclusively on his strong Vata characteristics for the sake of clarity. However Victor also has Pitta dosha as a secondary followed some way behind by Kapha. After working with Linda he consciously followed a Vata diet and all the practices that grounded his Vata tendencies and he made the changes necessary to alleviate his extreme Vata imbalances. Having nurtured his Vata dosha, always considering this first in the chain of cause and effect, it was likely that subsequent imbalances would come from his secondary dosha. He couldn't rule out Kapha imbalances but they would be less common than Pitta, which was stronger in him and closer to his primary dosha.

This was the case when, after several months, Victor started to have bouts of diarrhoea. Our digestive processes are great indicators of physical and emotional health. We cannot hide the effects of what goes on inside from ourselves, even if we are able to put on a public face to the world. Victor had learned that Pitta imbalances, arising as they do from fire and water elements, create anger and a tendency to challenge others, and in fact he had entered into a series of Pitta-like disagreements at work. If ever any anger cropped up in his life Victor was usually able to let it go quite quickly but for a period he found himself unable to let go of strong feelings of annoyance and exasperation at some of the antics of his colleagues. Normally he laughed off such feelings but now he had let things fester and kept going over them in his head long after the event. Without realising it his pulse would race and he would become flushed and hot. After a while he developed abdominal discomfort leading to diarrhoea, often the symptoms of IBS (irritable bowel syndrome), a typically hot Pitta complaint. Since heat was the keyword the remedy required immediate attention to his diet, with a reduction in all of the heating foods and spices, as well as the Pitta balancing ingredients of soothing music in a cool environment and walks in nature.

It would have been easy to put the diarrhoea down to a "tummy upset" and at that point many people might reach for the medicine cabinet and take a commercial remedy. Rather than do that Victor was able to recognise his problem by referring back to the list of qualities (Appendix H) and asking himself "What is the nature of this complaint?" He ran down the list ticking off each quality that corresponded with how he felt and selected hot, penetrating, sharp and slimy. From this he could take steps to sort out his problem. By identifying sharp Pitta pains he could treat his Pitta dosha in that moment with cooling food and spices; drinks such as aloe vera which would help to cool and flush out the Pitta; and using cooling cloths on his head that would help to calm the overheated temper he was trying to suppress. He could eat more root vegetables and Kichadi (a wholesome Ayurvedic dish) to cool and comfort his hot symptoms. Linda advised Victor to look at the reasons for his build up of anger; why, in this instance, was the balance tipped towards festering anger? Under scrutiny Linda found that Victor had other personal problems with his girlfriend and, romantically, things weren't going the way he wanted them to. These feelings had been playing on his mind and he hadn't been sleeping well; so a combination of these problems with the antics at work, had tipped the balance. Simply discussing it with Linda enabled Victor to release some of his inner angst.

Penelope was a predominantly Pitta dosha but with Kapha followed by Vata. She had worked with Linda's guidelines and for a long time was much better off from the effects of more suitable nutrition and the way she treated herself generally. She had begun to wear natural fabrics, had brought cooler colours into her home and took things slightly easier with her fitness workouts. Like Victor she had worked successfully with her primary dosha and was vigilant in addressing its needs, so any imbalances she experienced would be more likely to arise from her secondary Kapha dosha. Vata problems might also occur.

The stresses of her work never went away, but Penelope had learned to deal with them differently and was much more observant of her Pitta tendency towards anger and frustration with others. She had been on a more even keel emotionally and learned to behave calmly in situations that had previously caused her to flare up. This improved state of affairs lasted for some time despite increases in pressure; but then Penelope began to have headaches.

She could have had the typically piercing Pitta headaches she'd suffered with in the days before she met Linda, but these were different. They had a persistent, dull and throbbing kind of pain and when they came on they really shut down her normally lively personality. She felt like she was hearing and talking through a fog of low-key misery. She looked at the care she was taking with her Pitta dosha and there was nothing to indicate a problem.

She could have reached for the painkillers to mask the discomfort of a headache, but there was something else. At other times, despite her Pitta sparkiness Penelope began to suffer from bouts of lethargy. She would crash into periods of slothfulness and wouldn't look at things she normally dealt with immediately. She had periods when she behaved obsessively, focussing on negative trains of thought at one end of the scale, or the agenda for the extended holiday she was planning at the other end and during these low periods she felt apathetic and unable to cope. Her sleeping pattern would switch and she would be dead to the world. These were clear Kapha imbalances from her secondary dosha. To deal with these episodes Penelope needed to address Kapha excesses when they occurred. She looked through the list of qualities and noted that gross, heavy and slow seemed to describe how she felt and therefore indicated how to work with her complaint. When she was lethargic she needed to shift energy through conscious action. She would first need to look at the reasons why she felt shut down and unable to cope. Kapha excess often brings on a tendency to withdraw from events. Penelope should throw light on the problem by talking to a mentor or to friends and looking at any emotional issues she wasn't facing up to. She should take breaks and brisk walks to move energy that had become stuck and use eucalyptus inhalations and drink herbal teas with cardamom, ginger and a dash of lime to clear her head. Linda explained that Kapha lethargy is often due to overload and in this case it certainly seemed that Penelope was taking on too much.

Karen was a typical Kapha dosha, as we know, but she had a secondary Vata and minor Pitta dosha. She too had changed the way she looked after herself, her diet and many factors in her environment and as a result she felt livelier and was much more pro-active at work and in her recreational time. She increased her fitness levels through some long brisk walks and had even taken on the challenge of rugged mountain walks with new acquaintances. She felt re-vitalised and more decisive than she had done for some time. A social life had grown around the new activities and Karen found herself juggling agendas in ways she hadn't done before.

All was well but then Karen noticed changes to her skin condition. She had always been blessed with quite a good complexion and her naturally oily Kapha skin almost looked after itself, but she started to get dryness and flakiness on her face and around her hairline. Her hands became chapped and rough for the first time and her face became wind burnt face on her mountain days. She could have simply started to use different face cream to combat the skin problem but something else pointed to a better solution. She was thirstier than normal and found herself licking her lips a lot. This too could have been put down to too much talking and lots more exercise, but here is where knowledge of the qualities came in. She realised that dry, irregular and rough described her skin condition since the changes had shown up.

Dryness and thirstiness are all signs of a Vata imbalance and without realising it Karen had slipped into a Vata state because her newly vitalised social life and the increased exposure to sun, wind and rain tipped the balance within her doshas. Unfamiliar social pressures and the rigours of long mountain days placed demands on her metabolism. Karen was working and playing more energetically than ever before and the results materialised as Vata imbalance. Although Kapha types need to avoid too great an intake of fluid, Karen hadn't taken enough fluids to compensate for her increase in activity. She was eating lower fat food, fewer dairy products and more salads but the Vata imbalance created by the scope of her new interests had simply tipped the scales too far and she needed to look after her Vata dosha at that point. In addition, wind and sun had affected her, creating a Vata condition of roughness and dryness and she needed to use warm sesame oil for massage generally and for direct treatment to her face. Kapha types normally benefit from lighter oils but in this case she was working with a Vata condition which required Vata treatment. In Karen's case the imbalance did not come from an emotional problem, but from a change of activity.

In each case the diarrhoea, the headaches, the lethargy and the skin complaints were different forms of stress response. Stomach upsets do occur for all sorts of reasons, but Victor could plainly see that uncharacteristic behaviour on his part arose from pressure he experienced at work that he continued to re-cycle within his body, with the physical outcome displayed through his digestive tract. Headaches often result from an immediate response to pressured situations. Deadness and lethargy are depressive reactions to longer term stress levels. Just because Victor was a Vata type, he wasn't limited to Vata complaints, as we have seen. The same applied to Penelope and Karen. We normally exhibit the conditions of our primary dosha, but stress, nutritional problems and other factors can bring secondary and minor doshas to the fore and we need to be vigilant.

It is an odd fact but we often don't know how well we are until we're unwell! When our minds and bodies are in tune we run smoothly through the days and it's not easy to maintain vigilance because nothing interrupts our flow. Penelope's lethargy or headaches are good examples of the way a disturbance alerts us to a problem. Digestive upsets are good indicators of underlying conditions, and pain or discomfort should always be examined against the qualities.

Chapter 10

Simple Ayurveda Home Remedies

─────────

Many common complaints arise from disturbances in our doshas. They are manifested as discomforts, irritations, aggravations and dis-ease within the Qualities and Attributes (Appendix H), and can be relieved by working with herbal remedies.

Remember that Vata is cool and changeable, Pitta is hot and oily, and Kapha is cool and heavy. We can choose the remedy that will give the most benefit by considering these inherent qualities. Headaches are a frequent source of discomfort, but there are different kinds of pain. For example, someone with a burning headache will be experiencing a Pitta headache regardless of their dosha, and it's best to do something that cools the heat. Heavy, painful sinus pains indicate inflammation and congestion, which are Kapha conditions and it is best to relieve the congestion. In each case the underlying symptoms should be addressed in order to relieve the pain. Rather than take 'off the shelf' tablets, herbal remedies can act swiftly on the nervous system to alleviate and cure many complaints. These treatments have developed over hundreds and in some cases thousands of years and they are effective, natural and inexpensive.

Therapeutic Teas

One of the simplest and easiest ways to get instant therapeutic benefit from herbs and spices is to work with healing teas. Therapeutic teas benefit our bodies by speeding up the healing process. One of the most effective ways to take herbs is to drink them with water, which enables the energetics of the herbs to be taken directly into the system. This usually has an almost immediate effect, which is why these teas are so useful. They also taste good.

Depending on the herbs, spices and fruit used, therapeutic teas and be a wonderful part of your healing process during times of disease. Although therapeutic teas are often used to help us relax and sleep, they also have a much deeper healing job to do. Therapeutic teas can help during a programme of treatments; during convalescence; to give vitality; to reduce excess 'Pitta' heat; to improve the memory; to help as a weight reducing programme; to encourage bowel movement; to help insomnia; to cool down hot flushes; to clear toxins and to lift the spirits.

The main ingredients—herbs, spices and fruits—can be purchased locally from your health food shop, organic farm or even in the organic section of your supermarket. It is best to support your local small shops and farms, which provide an excellent service by giving us locally-grown products.

Ayurvedic Therapeutic Teas

There are two ways to work with herbal teas, described below. One uses the infusion process; the other uses the decoction process. We indicate which of these two processes should be used in the following list.

Standard infusion: 1 oz/25 grams *dried* herbs or 2 oz *fresh* herbs added to 1 pint/600 ml boiling water; or 1 tsp per cup. Leave to infuse for 5–10 minutes. Three to four cups a day.

Standard Decoction: Woody materials, roots, seeds and nuts, etc. Break down in a mortar and pestle. Same amounts as infusion, adding extra water to compensate for evaporation. Put into a pan cover with cold water. Bring to a boil, cover and simmer for 10–20 minutes max. Strain and drink—three to four cups a day.

Simple Chamomile Tea: One teaspoon of home-dried chamomile flowers can give more flavour than a commercial teabag. It is traditionally taken for irritable bowel syndrome, poor appetite, or indigestion. Drink a cup at night for insomnia, anxiety and stress.

Adding 200–400 ml strained infusion to a baby's bath water may help encourage sleep at night. Use as a standard infusion.

Cinnamon Tea: Cinnamon is good for all sorts of conditions, from the common cold to arthritis and rheumatism. The inner bark is usually used, mainly for digestive complaints including indigestion, colic and diarrhoea. It can stop vomiting and relieve flatulence. Also promotes sweating and can be used for treating colds. Use as a standard decoction.

Thyme and Elecampagne Tea: Thyme and elecampagne are two highly effective herbs for asthma which can be taken as teas or tinctures. Both are bronchiodilators and attack infection in the chest. Use as a standard infusion.

Oregano Tea: For soothing colic make a tea, leave to cool, and then strain the herb to leave a clear liquid. Feed the baby a little at a time. Try the same preparation for relieving coughs in adults. Additionally, to prevent or relieve a heavy chest cold, eat lots of oregano at key times. Hay fever sufferers may find some relief by sprinkling the dried herb on salads, and eating oregano in winter dishes can help loosen phlegm during the long months when common colds are prevalent. Use as a standard infusion.

Celery Seed Tea: May help prevent certain cancers, regulates blood pressure, and reduces cholesterol. Prepare a tea by pouring boiling water over one teaspoon of freshly crushed seeds. Let steep for 10 to 20 minutes before drinking. Use as a standard infusion.

Coriander Tea: Promotes digestion, eases colic, relieves arthritis, and prevents infection in minor wounds. Use one teaspoon of dried leaves or crushed seeds (or 1/2 teaspoon of powdered seeds) per cup of boiling water. Steep for five minutes. Drink up to three cups a day before or after meals. Weak coriander tea may be given to children under two for colic. You can also sprinkle the powdered seeds on minor cuts and scrapes. Before you do, thoroughly wash the wound with soap and water. Use as a standard infusion.

Dill Tea: Improves digestion, eases colic, fights flatulence, prevents infectious diarrhoea in children. To brew a stomach-soothing tea, use two teaspoons of mashed seeds per cup of boiling water. Steep for ten minutes. Drink up to three cups a day. To treat colic or gas in children under two, give small amounts of a weak tea. Use as a standard infusion.

Echinacea Tea: Fights infections, reduces symptoms of colds and flu, stimulates the immune system and heals minor wounds and burns. To make a tea, pour boiling water over two to three tablespoons of dried, fresh or powdered herb and steep for five minutes. Sip over a period of 30 to 90 minutes and repeat six to eight hours later. Use as a standard infusion.

Eucalyptus Tea: Eases congestion, relieves muscle soreness, and treats minor cuts. To brew a pleasant-tasting medicinal tea, use one to two teaspoons of dried, crushed leaves per cup of boiling water. Steep ten minutes. Drink up to two cups a day. Use as a standard infusion.

Fenugreek Tea: Minimizes symptoms of menopause, relieves constipation, controls diabetes, reduces cholesterol, soothes sore throat pain and coughs, eases minor indigestion, relieves diarrhoea. To make a medicinal tea, bring to a gentle boil two teaspoons of mashed seeds per cup of water, and then simmer for ten minutes. Drink up to three cups a day. To improve the flavour, you can add sugar, honey, lemon, anise or peppermint. Use as a standard decoction.

Ginger Tea: A traditional tonic; eases colds, soothes coughs, enlivens agni and promotes digestion. Add a teaspoon of fresh grated ginger, a teaspoon of honey, a squeeze of lemon to a cup of hot water.

Liquorice Tea: A traditional remedy; soothes sore throats, relieves coughs, heals peptic ulcers. Simply sprinkle a pinch of the powdered herb into hot water or tea. Unusually large amounts of licorice may cause stomach upset. If you find the drink doesn't agree with you, discontinue use.

Rosemary Tea: May prevent certain cancers, relieves menstrual cramps, aids digestion. Make a pleasant-tasting brew with one teaspoon of crushed dried leaves in a cup of boiling water. Let steep for ten minutes.

Lemon Balm & Tarragon Tea: Helps to heal herpes outbreaks, fights flu. Has antiviral qualities, lifts the spirits and is a good morning drink. For relief from either oral or genital herpes, try a cup of tea with a lemon balm tea bag and one teaspoon of dried tarragon. Let the brew steep for 10 to 15 minutes before drinking. Drink up to three cups a day. Use as a standard infusion.

Turmeric Tea: Turmeric aids digestion, relieves arthritis, treats dysentery, protects the liver, combats heart disease, wards off ulcers, prevents certain cancers. It tastes pleasant but in large amounts becomes somewhat bitter. To make a medicinal drink to aid digestion and possibly help prevent heart disease, use one teaspoon of turmeric powder per cup of warm milk. Drink up to three cups a day. Unusually large amounts of turmeric may cause stomach upsets. If you find the drink doesn't agree with you, discontinue use.

Rose Shatavari Tea—for women only: To 3 cups of water add 1 tsp dried organic rosebuds, 1 tsp shatavari powder and the juice of half a lemon. A nutritive and rejuvenating tonic. Cooling in energy with a sweet and bitter taste. Helps balance female hormonal system. Use as a standard infusion.

Ghee Tea: A soothing drink with mild anti-viral properties. To 3 cups of water add 1 tbs organic ghee and 1 tsp honey. Boil water then add ghee, let stand for a minute then add honey.

General Ayurvedic Skin Care

Our skin is the largest organ of our bodies and skin condition is a clear indicator of general health and of deeper problems. When we are well our skin glows when we are unwell our skin tone is dull, and poor complexion, rashes and inflammation can all occur.

The first and most important consideration with skin care is the Ayurveda Self Body Massage, which is recommended as a daily routine. For this we can use sesame oil, coconut oil or almond oil. Coconut oil is best for Pitta skins, sesame is best for Vata skins and Almond is a lighter oil and best for Kapha skin. We warm the oils, or in the case of Pitta keep at room temperature and massage our body from head to toe, keeping the oils on for as long as possible, even going to bed with them on if possible. The skin absorbs the oils, giving nourishment to inner tissues. The oils help our skin to feel supple and help strengthen the immune system. Self-massage draws our attention to the healing qualities of touch. Quiet attention to one's own body is an excellent way of bringing attention to the immediate moment and our own physical presence.

Aloe Vera is called 'kumari' meaning 'young maiden' in Sanskrit as it is used to help to keep skin looking young and vitalized. We advise clients to take Aloe Vera twice a day initially, morning and evening, to clear excess Pitta, which often shows as hot rashes on the skin. Once the complaint has subsided reduce the Aloe Vera. Drink with a little water or fruit juice and only use organic plant juice.

Sesame Oil. Linda tells all her clients to use sesame for many reasons; it is a nurturing, nourishing and healing heavy warm oil, especially good for dry skin, which benefits nervous or distressed people.

Rose Water is a wonderful tonic for the skin; Linda uses it with many clients as a cooling and refreshing skin drink. You can drink it and use it directly to tone and strengthen the skin cells. Pour a tablespoon in to your wash basin full of water every morning and rinse the face 10 times. To drink simply add a teaspoon to a glass of mineral water, and always buy organic. Rose water will immediately cool the skin and is great to have in a spray bottle to use when having hot flushes.

Neem is a bitter herb, which cleanses and has anti-viral qualities. It is an excellent herb for skin complaints and healing acne. Use neem soap or neem products from health stores to help keep acne at bay.

Orange peel, grated fenugreek and sandalwood are all good remedies for acne and skin complaints. Try using crushed orange peel; or make a paste using crushed fenugreek mixed with turmeric; or mix a paste of sandalwood and turmeric and use on the affected area.

As a general rule, to maintain good skin we should avoid greasy, excessively spicy and salty foods. Most skin problems indicate the lack of proper nutrition—and understanding your dosha will help you to balance any skin complaints. Also consider the following:

Water. Hydrate your skin everyday. Drinking adequate water helps to flush out toxins. Drink water according to your body type: Vata benefits most from lots of water; Pitta should drink water at room temperature, and Kapha should drink hot water with a heating tea. Remember that caffeine and alcohol are dehydrating, so drink more water if you drink a lot of tea or coffee.

Sleep. Sleep is crucial for tissue renewal and whole body health. See Chapter 6.

Exercise. Increases blood and lymph flow, encouraging the removal of toxins from the body. Exercise helps you to feel fit and more positive about yourself.

Exfoliate. Invigorate and cleanse your skin with a good skin care regime which involves exfoliation. Exfoliation cleans and prevents the clogging of pores and leaves the skin glowing and vital.

Smoking. Cigarette smoke contains toxins that actively damage your skin and also depletes the body of essential vitamins necessary for skin health, such as vitamin C and the B vitamins.

Headache Remedies

We have discussed headaches in relation to imbalances. They are painful, complex and commonplace, with a variety of causes but according to Ayurveda they come under the three dosha headings: Vata, Pitta, Kapha.

Vata headaches arise from fear, stress, nervousness, constipation, physical over activity and trying to do too many things at once. All of these can aggravate the Vata type person. The aggravation goes into the muscular, nervous and skeletal system causing Vata headaches, which tend to be at the back of the head area. These are characterised by throbbing, pulsating, migrating pain.

Whilst Vata types suffer from this type of headache most frequently all doshas can suffer from them. Vata headaches come with tension in the neck, shoulders, back, constipation and sciatica and get worse when we move around.

Remedies. Massage the neck, shoulders and upper back with sesame oil.

Massage feet and scalp with sesame oil.

Sesame oil drops in the nose.

Drink: mix 1 tablespoon sugar, quarter teaspoon salt, with lime or lemon juice in a pint of water.

Tea—using either ginger, rose flowers or basil.

Pitta headaches arise from acidity, hyperactivity, anger, aggression and indigestion, all symptoms of excess Pitta. The aggravation provokes headaches that are likely to be in the temporal area. Pain starts in the temple and moves to the centre of the head. Pitta headaches are sharp, shooting, burning, and penetrating pain. They become worse in bright light, under hot sun, after spicy foods, and in high temperatures. Pitta types become irritable and tend to get these headaches most frequently but all types can suffer from them. Eating sour, spicy food will make the pain worse. The headaches are related to the stomach area and sickness can be felt with burning stinging eyes.

Remedies. Cooling Aloe Vera gel taken in a drink helps cool the body.

Cool sweet food such sweet fruit or ice cream will help.

Coconut is cooling and soothing.

Tea—use cumin and coriander, or fennel, drink while still warm.

Kapha types **have sinus headaches**, which tend to be towards the front of the head. They are usually dull, deep and heavy and the pain moves into the sinuses. Kapha diets can create heaviness in the stomach which blocks circulation causing Kapha headaches. A Kapha headache gets worse when we bend down and is often connected to a stuffy nose, colds and coughs and also hay fever. Symptoms of lethargy and laziness accompany overeating, greed and possessiveness.

Remedies. Eucalyptus steam immediately helps to ease a Kapha headache.

Eucalyptus, lavender and tea tree oil massaged onto the forehead or inhaled in steam, or drops of oil on a handkerchief are all helpful.

Teas made from warming and spicy ginger and cinnamon provide relief.

Insomnia

A bad night's sleep is something we all experience occasionally but when it gets to be a regular occurrence it is often due to deeper, unresolved issues. Read Chapter 6 and consider the following suggestions:

- Remove salt from your diet—this is a stimulant.
- Avoid white flour and white flour goods.
- Avoid sugary canned drinks, alcohol, tea and coffee.
- Reduce fatty and spicy foods.
- Eat more whole grains and natural carbohydrates, pulses and nuts.
- Lack of physical exercise is another reason for general insomnia. Many people do not move from desks all day and travel to work in cars rather than walking.
- Dairy products are Kapha-based and have a calming effect; a pinch of nutmeg in a glass of warm milk can be helpful at bedtime.
- Practice meditation to calm the inner critic and consider what is creating the anxiety that keeps your mind on the go.

The Common Cold and Cough

The common cold and cough is a catarrhal and inflammatory condition of the upper respiratory tract caused by viral, allergic or mixed infections. In Ayurveda this is seen as aggravated Kapha, when the respiratory tract becomes congested creating a runny nose and a cough. There are many reasons for catching a cold but coughing usually increases in winter because people eat more-mucus forming foods like meat, sugar, white bread, porridge, puddings, etc. Coughing then creates airborne germs.

When the symptoms of a cold appears, Echinacea, Garlic and Elderberry are three herbs that can be combined to help to fight the virus and relieve respiratory discomfort.

A drink of cinnamon, cardamom, liquorice and black pepper flavoured with lemon and honey is effective in bringing relief from colds and flu.

Hot water with grated fresh ginger or honey helps to flush the system.

Eat warm, nourishing and easy to digest foods such as soups, grains and leafy green vegetables.

Cut down on foods and drinks that are mucous producing, such as dairy products and sugar.

Conclusion

Our bodies rebuild themselves many times throughout our lifetime, with cells from every organ renewed from the food that we eat. Every breath we take and every mouthful that we swallow contributes to this building process and to our existence. Every taste, every sight and smell, in fact every sensory experience connected with food rebuilds our cells. All that each cell needs is food that we get the pleasure of eating, and kindness, in the form of rest, exercise and thought.

The scary thing is that at the sub-atomic level there is very little that holds us together. Quantum science reveals that atoms and molecules are linked by little more than pulses of energy and when we look beyond these pulses, differences between apparently solid objects begin to vanish. We are in one sense less than we seem to be, and in another sense much more. Our bodies are composed of the five elements of earth, water, fire, air and space and all that we feel and do arises from this combination of elements and our resonating pulse of life. The quality of that pulse, the thoughts and actions that we put into our energy field become even more important when seen from this perspective.

We are not the body we inhabit, which is a temporary assembly of particles in a particular pattern. We are, in fact, that sustained pulse of energy, a life force and we share that characteristic with every other living creature. We vibrate at particular frequencies and we see and feel our world through the filter of these frequencies, which require maintenance, nourishment and care. Without that attention we lose awareness and the ability to feel. Without the ability to feel our emotions and all of the sensory messages that we receive, we become ever more closed and unable to receive and then unable to communicate our thoughts and true feelings.

We saw that Victor, Penelope and Karen had lost touch with themselves and continued to do things, eat things and think in ways that harmed them. That is what we all do for most of our lives. Now our three clients are aware of their inborn characteristics they can stop being victims and begin to take control, with genuine insight into their physical and emotional needs. This opportunity is open to all of us.

Appendices

Appendix A

Dosha Questionnaire

(Instructions: Read each series of statements horizontally, across each row and tick the statement(s) that apply to you. You may have more than one tick for each row, and that is OK, it simply means that you fall across two categories. You may want to ask a friend to help complete the questionnaire. Many people often find it difficult to be objective about their own bodies.

When you have worked through all the points go vertically down the columns, Vata, Pitta and Kapha adding up the number of ticks. You may then find, for instance, that you have 25 Vata, 18 Pitta and 10 Kapha. This would indicate you are a combined dosha of Vata/Pitta and you should eat and live your life to balance the dominant dosha.

You will see that our sub-headings include physical and mental traits, and you may need to take your emotional condition into account. For instance, you may have a Pitta imbalance that disguises the fact that you are more of a dominant Vata or Kapha type, or a dominant Kapha type may be suffering from Vata imbalances and so on. By balancing the predominant dosha revealed by the questionnaire you will relieve any temporary emotional imbalances.

It is advisable to repeat the questionnaire every three months to establish a clearer view of your dominant characteristics. Your underlying physical traits will not change and they are a reliable indicator of your dominant dosha, but other factors influence your emotional condition. A three monthly check will help maintain your awareness of any changes. Always balance the dosha that dominates at any given time.)

1 ~ Upper Body

Yourself	Vata	Pitta	Kapha
Body Frame	Thin, irregular, very short or very tall, bony, slender or rangy.	Medium, proportionate, toned, average frame.	Heavy, broad, stocky, stout, well developed.
Bones/Frame	Thin, small.	Average.	Large bones.
Joints	Small, cracking, prominent, dry, thin.	Medium, loose.	Large, well built.
Weight	Hard to gain weight, easy to lose, low, protruding veins and bones, fluctuating weight.	Easy to gain, easy to lose, moderate, muscular.	Easy to gain, hard to lose, heavy, tends to obesity.
Upper Body	Small, narrow, hard to gain weight, unproportioned.	Medium, well proportioned.	Large, well-developed, broad, gains weight easily.
Shoulders	Thin, flat, hunched.	Medium.	Strong, broad, thick.
Arms	Bony elbows, long, thin, small.	Average, wiry.	Big, heavy, well developed, fleshy.

Yourself	Vata	Pitta	Kapha
Fingers	Long, tapered.	Medium.	Short and squarish.
Nails	Small, thin, dry, rough, cracking, dark.	Soft pink, pliable, medium shape.	Wide, large, thick, white, smooth, firm.
Hands	Small, long, narrow, bony knuckles, cool, rough, dry.	Medium, warm, hot, sticky.	Large, solid, cool, square.

2 ~ Lower body

Yourself	Vata	Pitta	Kapha
Thighs	Thin, narrow, bony.	Medium proportion to body.	Cellulite, well developed, fat.
Legs	Thin, bony knees, very short or very long – co-ordination can be unsteady.	Averagely proportioned legs.	Stable, thick, stocky with standing power.
Calves	Slim, tight, wiry.	Medium proportion, soft, loose.	Large, shapely, firm.
Feet	Long or very small, thin, rough, dry, unsteady, long toes, cool.	Average size, soft pink, normal to warm, hot, sweaty.	Large, thick, steady, normally warm.

3 ~ Face and Head

Yourself	Vata		Pitta		Kapha	
Head	Long or small, thin, can be unsteady, can have stiff neck.	☐	Big, square, stocky, steady.	☐	Average, proportioned, steady.	☐
Hair	Curly/frizzy, dry, (brown), coarse, full head, split hair.	☐	Reds, blonde, straight, early grey, bald, soft and fine.	☐	Thick, wavy, dark, oily, shiny.	☐
Forehead	Small forehead with wrinkles.	☐	Average forehead with horizontal folds.	☐	Broad forehead and thick.	☐
Face	Small or long, thin and sallow, dull and wrinkles easily.	☐	Average shape, sharp contours, pinkish.	☐	Big, round, flattish, pale, soft features.	☐
Skin	Dry, cool, thin, rough, cracked, prominent veins. More difficult to sunburn.	☐	Warm, sometimes delicate and sensitive, pink, freckles, acne, moles, spots, rashes, easily sunburns.	☐	Cool, smooth, white, soft, moist, oily, fatty, good in the sun.	☐
Complexion	Dull, darkish without lustre.	☐	Flushed, freckles, glowing	☐	Pale.	☐

Yourself	Vata		Pitta		Kapha	
Eyes, Lashes and Brows	Eyes small, erratic, unsteady and prone to dryness. Lashes short and scanty. Brows large profuse or very small.	☐	Eyes medium, reddish, green, grey, piercing, light sensitive. Lashes moderate. Brows moderate.	☐	Eyes wide, oily, attractive, can cry easily, steady focus. Lashes lush, long. Brows strong.	☐
Nose	Thin, long or very small, pointed, dry, crooked.	☐	Average, pointed, sharp shape.	☐	Big, firm, oily.	☐
Lips	Narrow, small/large, dry, unsteady, dark.	☐	Medium, soft, red.	☐	Large, thick, oily, smooth, firm.	☐
Teeth and Gums	Small or large in size, crooked, rough, dry with spaces, protruding teeth, receding gums.	☐	Average proportioned teeth, gums soft pink that bleed easily.	☐	Big white square teeth, soft, pink strong gums.	☐
Mouth	Often dry with an astringent taste.	☐	Often salivating, with a bitter, pungent taste.	☐	Excess salivation, with sweet, salty taste and mucus in throat.	☐
Throat	Constricted throat, rough and dry throat.	☐	Sore, inflamed and burning.	☐	Swollen, tight.	☐

Yourself	Vata		Pitta		Kapha	
Stomach	Excess hiccupping, belching, variable appetite, feelings of constriction.	☐	Burning, sour, pungent belches or hiccups, excess appetite, heart burn.	☐	Sweet or mucus belching, slow digestion, feeling nauseous.	☐
Appetite	Variable, erratic, irregular, eats quickly, likes warm oily foods.	☐	Strong, sharp, intense, eats fast, enjoys cold foods.	☐	Low but constant, consistent, eats slowly likes warm, dry foods.	☐
Circulation	Poor, variable, palpitations, aggravated by wind, dry weather and the cold.	☐	Warm to hot, circulation good, aggravated by heat, fire and sun.	☐	Circulation slow and steady, aggravated by damp and cold.	☐
Tastes	Bitter, astringent and pungent.	☐	Sour, pungent and salty.	☐	Sweet, sour and salty.	☐

4 ~ Mental Traits

Yourself		Vata		Pitta		Kapha
Sensitivities	☐	Loud noise.	☐	Bright lights—strong sunlight	☐	Strong odours.
Voice/ Speaking	☐	Low, weak, whining, monotone, quick, talkative, rambling, imaginative—varied depending on changing moods.	☐	High, sharp, clear, precise, organized, detailed, orators, moderate, argumentative.	☐	Deep, tonal, singers, slow, silent, drawn out.
Dream/Sleep	☐	Flying, erratic, running, fearful, light sleep.	☐	Fighting, in colour, moderately deep, violent, intense.	☐	Romantic, water, few, heavy, deep sleep, long, watery.
Mind/Senses	☐	Fear, anxiety, apathy, sorrow, delusion, nervous, unconsciousness, insomnia, needing heat. Strongly dislikes cold things, loss of coordination, indecisive, perceptive.	☐	Violent, delirious, dizzy, fainting, needing cold, poor senses, intoxicated. Restlessness, heated head, impatient, hot tempered, critical, angry, arrogant, intelligent.	☐	Calm, lethargic, stupor, excessive sleep, slow perception, desires heat, dull, inert, greedy, stubborn, possessive.

Yourself	Vata	Pitta	Kapha
Memory/ Learning	☐ Quick to learn ideas but also forgets quickly, likes to study many things but becomes unfocused, learns by listening.	☐ Learns quickly, forgets slowly, focused, penetrating, dis-criminating, goal-oriented, learns best by reading and with visuals.	☐ Slow to learn but never forgets, learns by association, steady.
Nature	☐ Adaptable, quick, indecisive.	☐ Penetrating, critical, intelligent.	☐ Slow, steady, grounded, flat.
Memory	☐ Understands ideas quickly, then forgets quickly.	☐ Clear, sharp, quick and lasting.	☐ Slow to learn, but once learns, never forgets.
Faith	☐ Erratic, rebellious, changeable, spiritually disciplined.	☐ Leader, goals, fanatical, tendency toward material success.	☐ Loyal, constant, conservative, fundamentally material.
Emotions	☐ Anxious, nervous, fearful, changeable.	☐ Angry, irritable, argumentative, fiery.	☐ Content, calm, sentimental, slow to anger.
Habits	☐ Travel, culture, humour, eccentric, obsessive.	☐ Politics, sports, dance, competitive, determined.	☐ Water sports, flowers, cosmetics, business, lazy.

Yourself	Vata		Pitta		Kapha	
Mental Disorders	Anxiety attacks, hysteria, trembling.	☐	Rage, tantrums, excess temper.	☐	Depression, sorrow, lethargic.	☐
Life Pace	Fast, unsteady, erratic, hyperactive.	☐	Moderate, purposeful, goal-oriented.	☐	Slow, steady.	☐
Endurance	Low or fluctuating.	☐	Moderate to high, heat intolerance, pushes until one burns out.	☐	Strong, steady, slow starters, moderate performance.	☐
Sexual Nature	Variable, strong desire but low energy, cold.	☐	Moderate, passionate, domineering, quarrelsome.	☐	Constant, low, devoted, warm.	☐

5 ~ Symptoms of Disease

Yourself	Vata		Pitta		Kapha	
Initial Signs of Disease	Variable symptoms, irregular and rapid onset.	☐	High temperature/fevers, moderate onset.	☐	Slow but constant onset often from congestion.	☐

Yourself	Vata	Pitta	Kapha	☐
Disease Tendencies	Nervous disorders, immune system diseases, arthritic pains, mental disturbances, stress disturbances, bone and joint problems.	Infections, blood disorders, inflammation, yellow and green mucus.	Problems with respiratory disease, clear, white mucus, obesity.	☐
Disease Resistance	Poor resistance to disease, weak immune system.	Moderate resistance to disease, infections and bleeding.	Good resistance to disease, strong immune system.	☐
Healing/ Medicinal Requirements/ Tendencies	Heals quickly, requires low dosage, has nervous reactions.	Moderate—average.	Slow healing, requires higher dosage.	☐
Pain	Severe, sharp, disruptive, churning, throbbing, tearing, variable.	Moderate, burning, steaming, swelling, bleeding.	Mild, heavy, dull and constant.	☐
Fever	Variable, moderate heat, irregular, anxious and restless with a thirst.	High heat, burning thirst, irritable, delirious, sweating.	Low heat, constant, heavy and dull.	☐

Yourself	Vata	Pitta	Kapha
Discharges	☐ Gases—cracking joints, bones, sighing, moaning and groaning.	☐ Blood, yellow and green pus—aggressive, angry.	☐ Mucus, clear or white pus, salivation, quiet, lethargic.
Sweat/Odour Based On Daily Cleansing (Vegetarians sweat less than meat eaters)	☐ Odourless, scanty.	☐ Strong smell, profuse, hot.	☐ Pleasant smell, moderate when exercising, cold.
Faeces	☐ Scanty, dry, hard, painful, or difficult, gas, constipation.	☐ Abundant, loose, yellowish, burning diarrhoea. (Pitta persons with fevers get constipation.)	☐ Moderate, solid, pale, mucus in stool. (Kaphas may get constipation but stool is not hard.)
Urine	☐ Scanty, colourless, bubbly, difficult.	☐ Profuse, yellow, red, burning.	☐ Moderate, whitish, milky.

Appendix B
The Five Elements

Element	Dosha	Quality
Ether/ space	Vata	Light, mobile, cold and quick. Within the cool but creative potential of ether/space, Vata energy is transmitted quickly and without hindrance. Too much movement can occur, which is expressed as restlessness, and the inherent coolness of space needs to be guarded against.
Air	Vata	Dry, rough, irregular, cold and changeable. The passage of air can, like the wind, erode surfaces as it ebbs and flows shifting in strength and direction, always changing, never constant. It can freshen and bring life or it can enervate and sap energy.
Fire	Pitta	Light, hot, intense, sharp, penetrating, pungent and acidic. Fire provides the essential force for transformation and digestion of food, ideas and vital energy. By its very nature fire is hot and potentially sharp and intense, qualities that in excess can overpower, creating dryness, discomfort or damage.
Water	Pitta, Kapha	Medium and acidic, heavy, cold and smooth. Water flows to establish its own balanced level wherever it occurs, its natural weight providing the force to move all in its path yet also the basis for smooth, uninterrupted flow. Water is the medium in which transformative chemical reactions occur and can be tainted by unbalanced activity.

Element	Dosha	Quality
Earth	Kapha	Heavy, solid, stable, slow and structured. Earth is the grounding element, providing the level foundations upon which life can be built. Earth remains stable and relatively unmoving when other elements shift and transform, and most earth movement is slow when it occurs, like the tectonic plates of our planet's continents. Earth can become too heavy and immobile, like mud, at which point lethargy of body and mind occur.

Appendix C: **Vata Tastes: favour sweet, sour and salty**

Food type	Favour	Avoid
Dairy	All dairy in moderation, including buttermilk, cows milk, hard cheese, soft cheese, ghee, goats milk, goats cheese, ice cream, sour cream, yoghurt	Goats milk, all powdered milk products
Fruits	Sweet fruits: apricots, avocado, bananas, berries, cherries, coconut, dates, grapefruit, grapes, kiwi, lemons, limes, mango, oranges, peaches, pineapples, plums (sweet), raisins (soaked), rhubarb (sweet), strawberries	Apples, cranberries, dried fruits, pears, persimmon, pomegranate, prunes, quince, watermelon
Vegetables	Cooked vegetables: artichoke, asparagus, beetroot, carrots, courgettes, green beans (well cooked) leeks, okra, olives, onion, parsnips, potatoes (sweet), pumpkin, squashes. Salad: radish, cucumber, watercress	Frozen, dried or raw vegetables, artichoke, aubergine, broccoli, Brussels sprouts, cabbage, cauliflower, capsicums, celery, fresh corn, leafy greens, lettuce, mushrooms, raw onions, peas, potatoes (white), spinach, sprouts, tomatoes, turnips

Food type	Favour	Avoid
Beans/ legumes/ nuts/seeds	Beans in moderation; aduki, black lentils, mung, red lentils, soy cheese, soy milk, tofu, toor dhal. Nuts in moderation; almonds, brazil nuts, cashews, coconut, hazel nuts, macadamia nuts peanuts, pecans, pine, pistachio, walnuts. Seeds: Flax, sesame, pumpkin, and sunflower	All other beans; black beans, black-eyed peas, chana dhal, chick peas, kidney beans, brown lentils, lima beans, navy beans, pinto beans, soy beans, split peas, tempeh, white beans. Psyllium seed.
Grains	Oats (cooked), all rice, wheat, wild rice	Barley, buckwheat, cold, dry puffed cereals, corn, granola, millet, oats (dry), oat bran, quinoa, rice cakes, rye, wheat bran
Oils	All oils: almond, corn, coconut, canola, mustard, olive, sesame, sunflower	Animal fats and mixed vegetable oils
Spices	All spices; Ajwain, allspice, anise, asafoetida, basil, bay leaf, black pepper, caraway, cardamom, cayenne, cinnamon, cloves, coriander, cumin, dill, fennel, garlic (in moderation); ginger, mace, marjoram, mint, mustard seed, nutmeg, orange peel, oregano,	Horseradish, fenugreek, neem leaves, raw garlic

Food type	Favour	Avoid
continued	paprika, parsley, peppermint, poppy seeds, rosemary, saffron, sage, spearmint, star anise, tamarind, tarragon, thyme, turmeric, vanilla	
Summary	Favour warm, oily, heavy foods and sweet, sour and salty tastes. Use pungent, bitter and astringent tastes as accents, in moderation.	

Pitta Tastes: favour sweet, bitter, astringent

Food type	Favour	Avoid
Dairy	Unsalted butter, cottage cheese, mild soft cheese, ghee, cows' milk, goats' milk, ice cream, yoghurt (diluted)	Salted butter, hard cheeses, feta cheese, sour cream, yoghurt
Fruits	Sweet fruits; apples (sweet), apricots (sweet), avocado, berries (sweet), cherries (sweet), coconuts, dates, figs, grapes (sweet), mango, melons, oranges (sweet), pears, plums (sweet), pomegranate, prunes, raisins, watermelon	Sour fruit; apples (sour), apricots (sour), berries (sour), bananas, cherries (sour), cranberries, grapefruit, kiwi, lemons, limes, oranges (sour), papaya, peaches, pineapples, plums (sour), rhubarb, strawberries
Vegetables	Sweet and bitter vegetables; artichoke, asparagus, broccoli, Brussels sprouts, cabbage, capsicum, cauliflower, corn (fresh), courgettes, cucumber, celery, green beans, leafy greens, lettuce, mushrooms, okra, parsnip, peas, potatoes (sweet and white), squash, sprouts, watercress	Pungent vegetables; aubergine, beetroot, carrots, garlic, horseradish, leeks, olives, onions (raw and cooked), peppers (hot), pumpkin, radish, spinach, tomatoes, turnips

Food type	Favour	Avoid
Beans/ legumes, nuts/seeds	Aduki, black beans, black-eyed peas, brown lentils, chana dhal, chick peas, kidney beans, lima beans, mung beans, navy beans, pinto beans, soy beans, soy milk, soy cheese, split peas, toor dhal, tempeh, tofu, white beans. Coconut. Seeds: Psyllium, pumpkin, and sunflower	Black and red lentils, toor dhal. Almonds, brazil nuts, cashews, macadamia, peanuts, pecan, pine nuts, pistachio, walnuts. Flax seed, sesame seeds
Grains	Barley, oats (cooked), rice (Basmati and white), rice cakes, wheat, wheat bran	Buckwheat, corn, millet, oats (dry and bran), quinoa, rice (brown), rye
Oils	In moderation: avocado, coconut, olive, sunflower, sesame, soy, walnut	Almond, apricot, corn, sesame (dark)
Spices	Basil (fresh), black pepper (moderation), cardamom (moderation), cinnamon (moderation), coriander, cumin, dill, fennel, mint, neem leaves, orange peel (moderation), parsley (moderation), peppermint, saffron, spearmint, turmeric, vanilla	Ajwain, allspice, anise, asafoetida, basil, bay leaf, caraway, cayenne, cloves, fenugreek, garlic, ginger, horseradish, mace, marjoram, mustard seed, nutmeg, onion, oregano, paprika, poppy seeds, rosemary, sage, star anise, tamarind, tarragon, thyme
Summary	Favour cool food and liquids, sweet, bitter and astringent tastes and sour, salty and pungent tastes as accents	

Kapha Tastes: favour pungent, bitter, astringent

Food type	Favour	Avoid
Dairy	Low or non fat milk, low fat yoghurt (diluted), ghee (in moderation), goats' milk	All other dairy especially butter, cheeses, full cream milk, ice cream, yoghurt. See beans for soy alternatives
Fruits	Apples, apricots, berries, cherries cranberries, dried fruits and figs, peaches, pears, persimmon, pomegranate, quince, raisins	Sweet and sour fruits, avocado, bananas, coconuts, dates, fresh figs, grapefruit, (grapes and kiwi in moderation), lemons, limes, melons, oranges, mangos, papaya, pineapples, plums, rhubarb, watermelon
Vegetables	Raw, pungent and bitter vegetables, artichoke (in moderation), aubergine, asparagus, beets, broccoli, Brussels sprouts, cabbage, carrots, cauliflower, celery, corn (fresh) capsicum, garlic, green beans, horseradish, leafy greens, lettuce, mushrooms, okra, onions, parsley, potatoes (white, in moderation), spinach, sprouts, summer squash, turnips, watercress	Sweet juicy vegetables, cucumber, courgettes, olives, parsnip, sweet potatoes, pumpkin, tomatoes, squashes, sweet potato, swede
Beans/ legumes, nuts/seeds	Aduki, black beans, black-eyed peas, chana dhal, chick peas, lima beans, mung beans (in moderation) navy beans, pinto beans, red lentils, split peas—green or yellow, toor dhal,	Black lentils, kidney beans, brown lentils, soybeans, soy milk (cold), soy cheese, soy flour, tempeh, cold tofu. Almonds, walnuts, brazil nuts, cashew,

Food type	Favour	Avoid
continued	tofu (in moderation), white beans. (Flax, pumpkin, and sunflower seeds in moderation)	coconut, macadamia, peanuts, pecan, pine, pistachio nuts. Psyllium, sesame seeds.
Grains	Barley, buckwheat, corn, cornmeal, millet, oats (dry) oat bran, quinoa, basmati rice (in moderation), brown or white rice (in moderation), rye, wheat bran, wheat (in moderation)	Oats (cooked)
Oils	Almond, canola, corn, mustard, sunflower—all in moderation	Avocado, coconut, olive, sesame, walnut
Spices	Ajwain, allspice, anise, asafoetida, basil, bay leaf, black pepper, caraway, cardamom, cayenne, cinnamon, cloves, coriander, cumin, dill, fennel (in moderation), fenugreek, garlic, ginger (dry), horseradish, mace, marjoram, mint, mustard seed, neem leaves, nutmeg, onion, orange peel, oregano, paprika, parsley, peppermint, poppy seeds, rosemary, saffron, sage, spearmint, star anise, tarragon, thyme, turmeric, vanilla (in moderation)	Salt, tamarind, mango powder
Summary	Favour light, dry and warm foods and pungent, bitter and astringent tastes	

Appendix D
The Golden Section

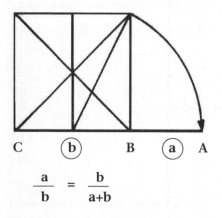

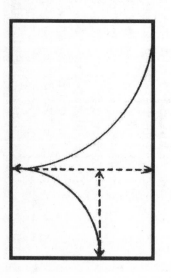

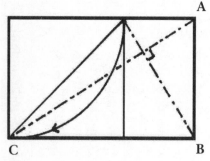

$$\frac{a}{b} = \frac{b}{a+b}$$

Mathematical systems of proportion originate from the Pythagorean concept that certain numerical relationships manifest the harmonic structure of the universe. One of these relationships has been in use since the days of the ancient Greeks and is the proportion known at the Golden Section. Temples, architecture and paintings since the Renaissance have used this proportion and it is impossible to escape its influences even today whenever ideas of harmony and proportion are involved.

The Golden Section can be defined as the ration between two sections of a line or the two dimensions of a plane figure 3 in which lesser of the two is to the greater as the greater is to the sum of both. This can be expressed algebraically thus:

A rectangle whose sides are proportioned according to the Golden Section is known as a Golden Rectangle. A square constructed on the smaller side of such a rectangle leaves a reaming portion that is a smaller version of the Golden Rectangle. This can be repeated indefinitely.

This progression closely follows the ration of the Fibonacci Series of numbers, (1, 1, 2, 3, 5, 8, 13, 21...) in which each number is the sum of the preceding two, relationships which continue to infinity.

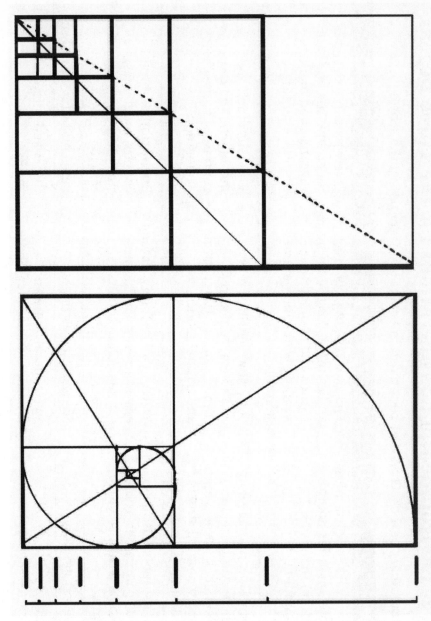

Diagrams illustrating additive and geometrical growth patterns based on the Golden Section. Check these proportions against classic photographs, paintings, page layouts, film scenes, architectural and civic spaces and landscape views.

Appendix E: Environmental Considerations for the Three Doshas

A summary of the factors that counteract imbalance and strengthen the senses

Senses	Vata	Pitta	Kapha
Sound	Classical music, running water, mantras, soothing natural sounds for grounding	Mantras, relaxing, cooling and calming classical music, hymns and choral music, running water and natural sounds	Lively rock 'n roll, last of the proms, the bustle of the street and markets, thunder, chanting
Touch	Firm, slow massage and touch; natural textures—wood, rock, fleeces and hats, sculptural structures and surfaces	Soft, slow, sensitive massage and touch, considered, meaningful contact; cotton and natural fabrics	Vigorous touch and movement and the contrast of light sensory exploration
Sight	Landscapes, seascapes, wide panoramas, cooler colours, visual arts in all forms	Water in all its forms, natural environments, landscapes, subtle cooling colours	Bright clothes, bright colours, rough seas, street life, sporting activity
Taste	Sweet, sour, salty	Sweet, bitter, astringent	Pungent, bitter, astringent
Smell	Earthy, sweet, floral, jasmine, sandalwood	Sweet, floral—rose and jasmine, vanilla, chamomile and lavender	Citrus and spicy herbal smells

Senses	Vata	Pitta	Kapha
Spirit	Meditation, peace and rest, stillness, cathedral, church and civic spaces	Meditation, cool fresh air, water and calm seascapes, churches	Brisk walks, social activity, windy mountain tops, chanting.

Appendix F
Three Part Breathing

This is one of the easiest and most profound breathing techniques that can be done anywhere at anytime. It promotes awareness, eases tension and enhances life force to the body.

1. Make yourself comfortable, seated or standing and take a deep breath, through the nose, into the abdomen, so that it expands out like a balloon.

2. On the next breath continue the inhalation from the abdomen and now expand the ribcage with air.

3. On the next breath continue to inhale from the abdomen and ribcage and now all the way to the upper chest, so it too expands like a balloon.

Reverse the procedure by exhaling out first from the chest, then the ribcage, and the abdomen, pulling in on the abdominal muscles at the end of the exhalation to remove all of the inhaled air.

Continue the process by breathing in again (Steps 1, 2 and 3).

Continue these repetitions for up to 15 minutes.

Appendix G
The Tilt of the Earth's Axis causes Seasons

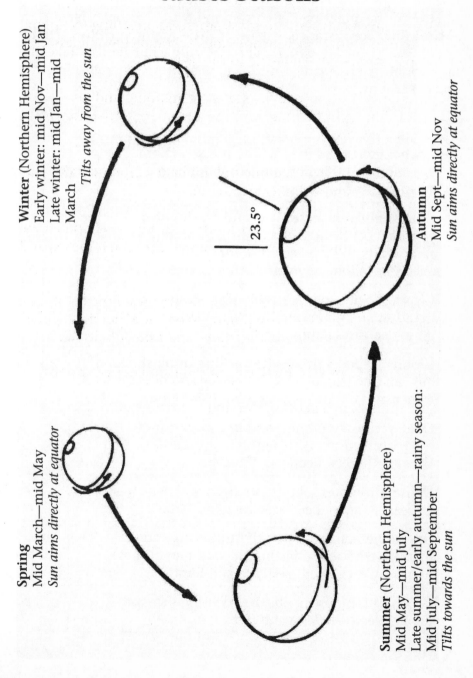

Winter (Northern Hemisphere)
Early winter: mid Nov—mid Jan
Late winter: mid Jan—mid March

Tilts away from the sun

23.5°

Autumn
Mid Sept—mid Nov
Sun aims directly at equator

Spring
Mid March—mid May
Sun aims directly at equator

Summer (Northern Hemisphere)
Mid May—mid July
Late summer/early autumn—rainy season:
Mid July—mid September
Tilts towards the sun

Appendix H
Qualities and Attributes of the Doshas

Use the right hand column to indicate which qualities have flared up. Count the qualities that correspond with those associated with each dosha. For instance, if you record 4 Kapha qualities, 2 Pitta and 1 Vata, you are experiencing a Kapha imbalance. Take the appropriate steps using nutrition, self-care and environmental considerations.

		Vata	Pitta	Kapha
1	**Acidic:** increases Pitta. Acidity is essential for digestion and transformation but damaging when present in excess.		•	
2	**Changeable:** increases Vata and can involve considerable confusion and discomfort and an inability to be precise, but for Kapha can encourage momentum and movement.	•		
3	**Clear:** pacifies and cleans but also creates isolation and diversion. Increases Vata and Pitta, decreases Kapha.	•	•	
4	**Cloudy:** reduces penetrating acidity or harshness but can also lead to a lack of perception or clarity. It increases Kapha, decreases Vata and Pitta.			•
5	**Cold:** creates numbness and unconsciousness, fear, contraction and insensitivity. Increases Vata and Kapha, decreases Pitta.	•		•
6	**Dense:** promotes solidity, strength and density. Increases Kapha, decreases Vata and Pitta.			•
7	**Dry:** increases absorption of fluids, can lead to increased dryness, constipation and nervousness. Increases Vata, decreases Pitta and Kapha.	•		
8	**Gross:** causes obstruction and obesity. Increases Kapha, decreases Vata and Pitta.			•

	Vata	Pitta	Kapha
9 **Hard:** increases strength and hardness but also rigidity, selfishness, callousness and insensitivity. Increases Vata and Kapha, decreases Pitta.	•		
10 **Heavy:** increases bulk and mass but can cause dullness, lethargy, heaviness. Increases Kapha, decreases Vata and Pitta.			•
11 **Hot:** promotes heat and good digestion, cleansing and expansion, leads to inflammation, anger and hate. Increases Pitta, decreases Vata and Kapha.		•	
12 **Intense:** can be both active and passive, increases Vata and Pitta and provides energy to Kapha.	•	•	
13 **Irregular:** increases Vata and creates confusion because of the element of unpredictability.	•		
14 **Light:** helps digestion, reduces bulk cleanses, creates freshness, alertness; leads to ungroundedness. Increases Vata and Pitta, decreases Kapha.	•	•	
15 **Liquid:** promotes salivation and cohesiveness, dissolves and liquefies. Increases Pitta and Kapha, decreases Vata.		•	•
16 **Medium:** epitomizes the essence of balanced Pitta attributes.		•	
17 **Mobile:** promotes motion and also movement, restlessness and lack of faith. Increases Vata and Pitta, decreases Kapha.	•	•	
18 **Oily:** creates smoothness, moisture, movement, lubrication, vigour but in excess causes ingratiating, manipulative behaviour. Increases Pitta and decreases Vata and Kapha.		•	
19 **Penetrating:** increases Pitta and is often experienced as a piercing sensation.		•	

	Vata	Pitta	Kapha
20 **Pungent:** increases Vata and Pitta and is the hottest and driest quality, thus decreasing Kapha.	•	•	
21 **Quick:** increases Vata and Pitta and decreases Kapha,and since it is the opposite of slow it can create aggravation.	•	•	
22 **Rough:** causes cracking of the skin and bones and creates carelessness and rigidity. Increases Vata, decreases Pitta and Kapha.	•		
23 **Sharp:** promotes sharpness, quick understanding of information and situations, quick effect on the body; ulcers and irritation (skin, stomach, intestines, eyes and general disposition. Increases Vata and Pitta, decreases Kapha.	•	•	
24 **Slimy:** decreases roughness and increases smoothness and care. Increases Pitta and Kapha, decreases Vata.		•	•
25 **Slow:** creates relaxation and slow action, increases sluggishness and dullness. Increases Kapha, decreases Vata and Pitta.			•
26 **Smooth:** increases Kapha and is connected to body movement, skin condition and speech.			•
27 **Soft:** creates softness, delicacy, tenderness, relaxation and care. It increases Pitta and Kapha and decreases Vata.		•	•
28 **Solid:** increases Kapha and is connected to body movement, skin condition and speech.			•
29 **Stable:** a Kapha quality that, in excess, can become inflexible but stability is a positive trait that centres body and mind.			•
30 **Static:** promotes stability, support and faith but also leads to obstruction and constipation. Increases Kapha, decreases Vata and Pitta.			•

	Vata	Pitta	Kapha
31 **Structured:** a Kapha trait that is beneficial to both Vata and Pitta.			•
32 **Subtle:** penetrates the capillaries and increases feelings and the experience of emotions. Increases Vata and Pitta, decreases Kapha.			•

Ayurvedic Resources

UK and Europe

Ayurveda Clinic and Academy
Raddon House
641 Knutsford Road
Latchford Village, Warrington
Cheshire, WA4 1JQ
Tel: +44(0) 870 750 8363
Tel: + 44(0) 1925 652435
Email: info@ayurvedaclinicandacademy.com
Website: www.ayurvedaclinicandacademy.com
*Authentic Ayurveda treatments, diagnosis, nutrition, cooking and
training. The authors of 'Dosha for Life'.*

Ayurveda Practitioners Association
106 Whitchurch Gardens
Edgeware
Middlesex, HA8 6PB
Website: www.apa.uk.com

European Institute of Vedic Studies
Ayurvedic education
B.P. 4, 30170 Monoblet,
France
Website: www.atreya.com

USA

National Ayurvedic Medical Association
620 Cabrillo Avenue
Santa Cruz, CA. 95065
Tel: + 1-800 669-8914
Website: www.ayurveda-nama.org

American Institute of Vedic Studies
Dr. David Frawley
P.O. Box 8357
Santa Fe, NM 87504
Website: www.vedanet.com
Tel: +(1) 505-983-9385
Email: vedicinst@aol.com

The Ayurvedic Institute
Dr. Vasant Lad
P.O. Box 23445
Albuquerque, NM 87192-1445
Tel: + (1) 505-291-9698
Website: www.ayurveda.com

Ayurvedic Veterinary Associations

American Holistic Veterinary Medical Association
Website: www.ahvma.org/
The organization supports the study of many types of botanical medicine, including Ayurvedic. The organization states:"Herbs have healing powers that are capable of balancing the emotional, mental and physical dimensions of animals."

Veterinary Botanical Medical Association
Website: www.vbma.org/
VBMA is dedicated to promoting responsible herbal practice by encouraging research and education, strengthening relations with the industry, keeping herbal traditions alive as valid information sources, and increasing professional acceptance of herbal medicine for animals. The association also emphasizes herbal-drug interactions that may help or hinder the outcome of treatment. This site contains studies of the effect of many commonly used Ayurvedic medications, including aloe, boswellia, fenugreek, garlic, ginger, licorice, neem, pepper, tea tree, turmeric, and modern herb combinations. The organization also publishes a journal.

Sources for Ayurvedic Herbs and Products

Your local health food store may offer Ayurveda herbs, supplements, and oils, but you can also purchase them online from many organic and Ayurvedic sources including:

Ayurveda Clinic and Academy
Website: www.ayurvedaclinicandacademy.com

Ayurveda
Website: www.ayurveda-herbs.com/

The Ayurveda Center
Website: www.holheal.com/ayurved4.html

The Ayurvedic Institute
Website: www.ayurveda.com/products/ayurvedic_herbs.html

Ayurveda Marketplace
Website: www.ayurveda-herbal-remedy.com/herbal-
                  encyclopedia/

Ayurvedic Cure
Website: www.ayurvediccure.com/

Ayurvedic Herbs Direct
Website: www.ayurvedicherbsdirect.com/

Banyan Botanicals
High quality herbs and tinctures
Website: www.banyanbotanicals.com/

Herbs Forever
Website: www.satveda.com

Himalaya Herbal Healthcare
Website: www.himalayahealthcare.com/
Natural Herbs Guide
Website: www.naturalherbsguide.com/ayurvedic-herbs.html

Pukka Herbs
High quality herbs and tinctures.
Website: www.pukkaherbs.com

Organic Herb Trading Company
Organic herbs and tinctures
Website: www.organicherbtrading.com

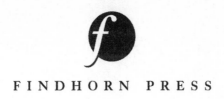

FINDHORN PRESS

Books, Card Sets,
CDs & DVDs
that inspire and uplift

For a complete catalogue,
please contact:

Findhorn Press Ltd
305a The Park, Findhorn
Forres IV36 3TE
Scotland, UK

Telephone +44-(0)1309-690582
Fax +44-(0)1309-690036
eMail info@findhornpress.com

or consult our catalogue online
(with secure order facility) on
www.findhornpress.com